T0323140

CULTIVATING YOUR
MICROBIOME

"Finally! A book demonstrating how the ancient traditional medical systems of both China and India understood the importance of the gut microbiome. The ancients, along with Hippocrates, declared that all diseases begin in the gut. As part of both the digestive and immune systems, numerous health problems result once these delicate flora are disturbed: autoimmune diseases, food allergies, and cancer, to name a few. Reestablishing intestinal health should be the starting point for the treatment of any disease. The research cited throughout this book corroborates over and over what these ancient doctors described in their texts thousands of years ago. A must-read for anyone interested in getting to the root cause of all diseases."

MARIANNE TEITELBAUM, D.C., AUTHOR OF
HEALING THE THYROID WITH AYURVEDA

"As a practitioner of Ayurveda and Chinese medicine, I loved how Bridgette wove these amazing systems of healing with our modern understanding of the microbiome. *Cultivating Your Microbiome* is a wealth of information and practices that will absolutely serve the seasoned health practitioner. Remarkably, it is also a book that can be read by anyone interested in improving their health and understanding the underlying principles of real well-being. *Cultivating Your Microbiome* is a must-read for all health practitioners and enthusiasts alike."

JONATHAN GLASS, M.AC, AYURVEDIC PRACTITIONER
AND AUTHOR OF *TOTAL LIFE CLEANSE*

"A fascinating book on the microbiome! *Cultivating Your Microbiome* combines the recent Western scientific knowledge and the teaching of the several millennia-old Eastern medicines."

CHRISTOPHER VASEY, N.D., AUTHOR OF
THE ACID–ALKALINE DIET FOR OPTIMUM HEALTH

CULTIVATING YOUR
MICROBIOME

Ayurvedic and Chinese Practices for a Healthy Gut and a Clear Mind

BRIDGETTE SHEA, L.Ac., MAcOM

Healing Arts Press
Rochester, Vermont

For my daughter, Calliope,
and all of her good critters

Healing Arts Press
One Park Street
Rochester, Vermont 05767
www.HealingArtsPress.com

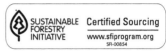

Text stock is SFI certified

Healing Arts Press is a division of Inner Traditions International

Copyright © 2020 by Bridgette Shea

All rights reserved. No part of this book may be reproduced or utilized in any form or by any means, electronic or mechanical, including photocopying, recording, or by any information storage and retrieval system, without permission in writing from the publisher.

Note to the reader: *This book is intended as an informational guide. The remedies, approaches, and techniques described herein are meant to supplement, and not to be a substitute for, professional medical care or treatment. They should not be used to treat a serious ailment without prior consultation with a qualified health care professional.*

Cataloging-in-Publication Data for this title is available from the Library of Congress

ISBN 978-1-62055-780-8 (print)
ISBN 978-1-62055-781-5 (ebook)

Printed and bound in the United States by Lake Book Manufacturing, Inc. The text stock is SFI certified. The Sustainable Forestry Initiative® program promotes sustainable forest management.

10 9 8 7 6 5 4 3 2 1

Text design and layout by Priscilla Baker
This book was typeset in Garamond Premier Pro with Museo Sans and Gill Sans used as display typefaces
Illustrations by Deborah J. Neary

To send correspondence to the author of this book, mail a first-class letter to the author c/o Inner Traditions • Bear & Company, One Park Street, Rochester, VT 05767, and we will forward the communication, or contact the author directly at **www.bridgetteshea.com.**

Contents

PART I

Modern Science Meets Ancient Wisdom

PART 2

Practices for Daily Living

Preface

As I put the finishing touches on this book, we are in the midst of the coronavirus pandemic. Last winter, when I first heard a report about a new pneumonia virus in China, I knew that this was going to be bad. I found out everything I could about it. One of the things I have enjoyed most about writing this book, as well as one of its greatest challenges, is how every single day there is new information being published about the microbiome, some of it even contradicting previously accepted truths. This virus is no different. Information on it changes daily, multiple times a day even. Like the microbes that make up our microbiomes, it is everywhere and it affects every human on the planet, directly or indirectly.

As I sat down to write this preface, I asked myself, *What is it that I need to tell my readers?* Unlike other times when I have asked a question and allowed space for inspiration to arrive, it took only a moment for the answer to come. I want my readers to know how to do something fundamental, something totally different in terms of how they view the body, pathogens, medicine, prevention, and healing. This is something that microbiome science will evolve to make us do. It is what Eastern medicine already does, and it is this: It cultivates our internal environment. My primary message here is to encourage you to recognize your body as part of nature and learn how to tune in to and take care of it in an effort to cultivate your microbiome. Eastern medical traditions focus on cultivating the internal landscape: tilling, weeding, and fertilizing the inner soil of our mucosa and tissue terrains using medicinal substances, foods, and lifestyle guidance geared toward living in harmony with nature and its cycles.

That is what this book is about. That is what treating people infected with coronavirus or any other pathogen is about. We in the Western world could have done better helping people suffering from this virus, and we still can—by utilizing the wisdom and herbal medicine of the Chinese medical tradition. Did you know that the Chinese government officially promoted traditional Chinese medicine for prevention and treatment of COVID-19? Or that it is being used alongside Western medicine in Chinese hospitals? Do you even know what traditional or classical Chinese medicine is? So many people have beliefs that anything from China is bad. They are afraid of Chinese herbs. Maybe they think Chinese medicine is just acupuncture and animal parts. This set of beliefs could be preventing these folks, and others who don't subscribe to them, from accessing the heart and soul of the medicine: the medicinals themselves.

In researching this virus, I have spent hours and days and weeks and now months following what is being done in China, with Chinese medicine, to help people. Those in the hospitals in Hubei province, where Wuhan is, are receiving Chinese medicine alongside Western treatments. The Chinese herbal decoctions they are receiving are bringing down fevers when the Western medicines are failing. They are helping people get out of the hospital faster and breathe fresh air again. How are they doing this? By supporting the body's inner terrain. These medicines are helping the body clear the fluids that build up, the dampness, and making the person's body a less habitable environment for the pathogen. These medicines are cultivating the individual's inner ecosystem to not only help the body in a state where it is overwhelmed, helping to balance the inflammatory and immune responses, but also to help the body clear the virus and any potential opportunistic coinfections. These medicines are also mitigating the side effects of Western drugs.

There are memes circulating on the internet about the formula the Chinese are using and many people are asking me about this herb or that. There is no one formula. There is no one herb. Do you make a pasta dish with just wheat? Do you bake a cake with only eggs? Do you fertilize soil with only carbon? The environment in every person's body is different. The inner landscape is different. The amount of fluids, dryness, heat, and cold are different. The strength of the body, the stamina, the immune function, the microbiomes are all completely different. Our microbes live in very specific environments. I often say that the health and diversity of the digestive tract microbiome is dependent upon whether or not we have a "Goldilocks gut": not too hot, not too dry, not too cold, not too acidic, not too oxygen-rich here or carbon dioxide-rich there, but *just right*. Chinese herbal medicines and Eastern medicines and lifestyle guidance are designed to make that Goldilocks gut happen.

This is why Chinese herbs are helping people recover from this coronavirus disease, and why they are endorsed by the Chinese government for treatment and prevention. And because no two inner terrains are alike, no two ecosystems are alike, wherever possible these formulas are being modified to match what the patient needs in each moment. This pathogen is shifty; it changes and appears to ebb and flow. People are presenting with the gamut of symptoms—from upper to lower respiratory, fever to no fever, sore throat or not, to digestive complaints. This pathogen is illustrating like none other in the collective consciousness just how environment-dependent its action is.

Why it generally spares children is also a mystery. I've heard a myriad of rationales behind it, but I'm wondering how much it has to do with the childhood gut microbiome. The gut flora of a child under nine years old is much different than that of a teen or an adult. One thing that sets it apart is the amount of bifidobacteria it contains. Bifidobacteria support immunity and help keep the gut wall intact. In infants, especially those who are breast-fed and delivered vaginally, the gut microbiome contains at least 60 percent bifidobacteria, as opposed to less than 10 percent in the adult gut.

These differences in the gut microbiome also almost certainly have something to do with the statistics of older adults and immuno-compromised people succumbing more to the virus—getting harsher cases of COVID-19 and even dying. As you'll learn in this book, a diverse microbiome is considered a healthy microbiome. Science is still catching up when it comes to how the individual's environment—what we describe as doshas, environmental factors, humors, elements, and constitution—is the bedrock of diversity. So far, science has found that the microbiome changes for the worse as we age, and that those with autoimmune conditions and various other "underlying health conditions" house less diverse microbiomes. Since the microbiome has a direct relationship to immune function, this is no surprise. In Eastern medicine we never overlook the state of the gut when looking at any person, regardless of what pattern or disease state they are presenting with. In fact, balancing the digestion and the ecology of the gut is a primary focus in treating not only most pathogens but any pattern of disharmony, or illness, in general.

Whether or not gut symptoms are a primary complaint, the ancients recognized that without its proper nourishment and function, we're done. They may not have had a word for the microbiome, but they knew of it and treated it as they saw it. Chinese medicinal herbs are classified according to taste and microbes respond to tastes and act accordingly. Microbes even regulate each other, sometimes based on flavor inputs, which you'll see by example later in this book. The information contained in an herb formula will activate or inactivate microbes and their processes as well as human cell functions. The information contained in herbal medicines increases or decreases circulation; directs how energy, blood, and fluids flow; builds tissues or degrades substances; regulates the inflammatory response; feeds the beneficial microbes that crowd out pathogens; changes the internal environment; creates mental clarity; balances the nervous response; and supports immunity, just to name a few things.

If you're on the fence about Chinese medicine, know that practitioners are incredibly well trained in wisdom that goes back thousands of years. In modern times, this wisdom is transmitted in extremely intensive, state accredited clinical training programs. In the United States, licensed Chinese medicine practitioners have completed an average of seven to eight years of undergraduate and postgraduate study, passed a national board exam, and received state licensure. Chinese medicine students do internships in Western medical facilities and spend hundreds, often times over a thousand, hours treating clients and using herbs under the guidance of extremely experienced clinicians—learning contraindications, drug interactions, and herb-herb interactions. In Tibet and as extensions of Tibetan programs abroad, practitioners are trained for four to five years. And in India Ayurvedic doctors are trained for a total of seven years. In China many hospitals have a traditional medicine wing so that both Eastern and Western medicines may be integrated on site. Although acupuncture is also being used in hospitals in China, and some in the West, acupuncture and Chinese herbal medicine are actually two different disciplines. Traditional or classical Chinese medicine is more focused on the herbs and medicinals used for cultivating the body's environment; it is internal medicine.

If you're trained in Eastern medicine, I urge you to promote it. We may have missed the boat on helping people with this first wave of novel coronavirus, but let it be a lesson to us as skilled health practitioners for the future. Forget the arguments that patients are noncompliant and won't take their herbs, or that they just want acupuncture. When people understand the importance of the Goldilocks gut, of cultivating their internal terrain and microbiomes—as they will learn to do over the coming years—they will take their herbs. Spread the word about Eastern medicine now, before the next wave of coronavirus, or whatever, comes down the pike. Do it for when we are in the space between dystopian times, when we have the luxury of focusing on leaky guts and chronic and autoimmune conditions. Educate your patients, contact your news agencies, urge your state organizations to push for widespread acceptance and education of the public about Chinese, Tibetan, and Ayurvedic medicines. Do this now while we can. We know the power of this medicine like no one else. It's our responsibility—to the medicine, to our fellow human beings, and to ourselves and our integrity as medical practitioners—to promote our medicine.

Acknowledgments

To my muse, Calliope, who doesn't like me to go to work but never protested when I needed to spend time writing. To her father, Nathan Solomon, who encouraged me throughout this process, knowing how grueling it can be, even to the detriment of time that could have been spent together. To my parents, who have always encouraged me to follow my path, regardless of whether or not I was bushwhacking. To Trisha LaPolt, Calliope's Bubbe and my dear friend, for her unending support. To Karen Carey, an amazing coach, and friend, for all of her support and help during this process. To Pernille Dake, who encouraged me just when it was needed. To Joe Kulin, "the great connector," for making this possible. To Deborah Neary, for her willingness, patience, and focus, and her wonderful artwork. To Jon Graham, who had great enthusiasm for this idea and without whom this book wouldn't have happened, as well as the entire Inner Traditions staff. To Lama Lhanang Rinpoche, whose magical nature created the space for this process to unfold. And to every person who walked through the doors of the Ageless Acupuncture clinic and asked me how the book was going. Your encouragement, support, and advice are a part of this work and I am forever grateful.

The Fascinating World
of Microbes

The human gut microbiome is likely the hottest scientific topic trending right now. Even those who don't know the word *micro-biome* are aware of what's called the gut-brain connection, or the second brain in the gut, and the existence of probiotics. Some may not even know the word *probiotics,* but will recognize brand names containing what are believed to be beneficial bacteria residing in the gut, and know that certain yogurts contain something said to help the gut as well. What most people may not know is the extent to which scientists are discovering the diverse roles that our inner microbial colonies play in keeping us healthy and happy.

We are emerging from a paradigm in science and medicine that has held the belief that microbes are bad, dirty, or dangerous. Swedish botanist Carl Linnaeus, the first to classify microbes in Western science, categorized bacteria under the genus *Chaos*.[1] I specify that he was the first to classify them in Western science, because in Eastern medicine, they and their genes and metabolites have been referred to for thousands of years under various names. We are at the cusp of a new paradigm, or perhaps just the renaissance or revival of an old one, in which the other half of the story on microbes—that they have a good, necessary, beneficial role to play—is finally emerging.

So, what is a microbe? According to David R. Montgomery, Ph.D. and Anne Biklé, authors of *The Hidden Half of Nature,* a microbe is any microorganism smaller than a millimeter,[2] and microbes are responsible for half the weight of living matter on Earth.[3] They are everywhere and eat pretty much anything. They exist in unexpected places, including cloud droplets in the upper atmosphere[4] and caustic hot springs in Yellowstone National Park. On our bodies they collectively weigh a few pounds. The gut microbiome actually weighs about as much as the brain, which is generally close to three pounds in an adult human. There is roughly a 1:1 split between our human cells and our microbial inhabitants.[5] This means that for every human cell in us, there is a microbe. These microbes include bacteria, viruses, archaea, fungi, and yeasts. I suggest we look at what Eastern medicine practitioners call *qi* or *prana*—what I call "vitality"—as containing microbes that positively influence our minds and bodies. In the Chinese tradition, "evil qi," which encompasses the six pernicious influences, or pathogenic factors, of wind, cold, heat, summerheat, dryness, and dampness, may include— and may actually *be*—harmful microbes, such as the flu virus. Eastern teachings also include words to describe microbes. Chinese medicine uses the word *chong,* which is translated as "bug." Ayurveda refers to *krimi,* or worms, and includes intestinal parasites that are visible to the naked eye, such as pinworm, hookworm, tapeworm, and roundworm; or invisible but recognizable by the signs and symptoms of the infected individual.[6]

Gut flora, or the microbial gut organ, is responsible for more than we scientifically know at this point, and what we do know about how it works is both overwhelming and limited. It is overwhelming in that there is a constant stream of new information about it daily. This information contains insight into previously unidentified strains, the workings of the strains we are familiar with, how they interact with one another, and how they affect us. All of this information, and the knowledge that certain states are linked to specific microbiome changes or patterns, raises questions about what a healthy microbiome is, what an unhealthy microbiome is, and potential treatments that may be developed in the future. In terms of the human microbiome, scientists admit that at this point they are just beginning to grasp not only who the key microbial players are, but also how they may balance, work with, or operate in opposition to each other.[7] This makes our overwhelming wealth of knowledge about the microbiome feel limited because we don't actually know enough scientifically to use it for healing. We can grasp the microbiome's potential for curing and preventing disease, but as of yet there are not many developed treatments other than fecal microbiota transplantation (FMT), and limited access even to that.

What we do know is that there is a gut-brain axis through which the gut microbiota—meaning all the microorganisms in the gut—affect moods and overall mental and emotional life, as well as almost all of our bodily functions. The gut microbiome influences our immune function, hormonal balance, cravings, sleep, inflammatory response, digestion, assimilation, and elimination. It breaks down substances we otherwise would be unable to digest and converts them into usable products. Our microbes help our bodies grow; have a molecular "nose" that smell toxins in the environment; break down toxins, including environmental chemicals; and not only make it difficult for bad microbes to thrive, but help to destroy them. They produce vitamins and minerals, for example, B12, and neurotransmitters such as serotonin. They train our immune system, help it recognize beneficial microbes as harmless to the body, help develop the nervous system, and influence our behavior.[8] They even play a role in how we respond to vaccines and other therapies.[9]

As if things aren't sounding complicated enough, it is not just the microbes themselves we are researching, but their genes, the surface molecules they carry, and the products or metabolites they produce. The gut microbiome alone produces hundreds of thousands of metabolites.[10] In fact, many researchers now refer to the microbiome as an organ.[11] The results from a recent fecal transplant—a process whereby feces are transferred from a healthy donor to a recipient needing healthy bacteria—were so astounding that one scientist likened it to an organ transplant. As Ed Yong notes in his bestseller *I Contain Multitudes,* "This makes the microbiome the only organ that can be replaced without surgery."[12]

What's even more amazing is that the microbiome can switch on genes that, for example, create blood vessels or aid in nutrient absorption. Because of this gene interplay, it has an impact on our genetic expression and whether or not predispositions manifest as our reality, and it is not always a favorable reality. The microbiome may adversely affect our genes after a major life stressor, for example, by flipping the switch that activates the gene for celiac disease.

In addition to the "good" bacteria in the gut making our lives more livable, we also have "good" viruses and fungi. No longer can we look at bacteria and viruses only as evils to protect against, as self vs. other. Now we know self is also other, and whether we knew it or not, we need both.

Do you remember being taught in introductory biology that mitochondria, the so-called "powerhouses" of the cell, were ancient bacteria that evolved into organelles—specialized subunits within cells? I do. I remember how unsettling it felt to learn that a major part of me was actually ancient bacteria. Recent studies show the long-accepted mitochondria succession is questionable, but the fact remains that our mitochondria did evolve from a proteobacterial lineage. In addition, genetic information we carry may be ancient virus data we have assimilated into ourselves. This revelation that as our species has evolved we've assimilated what we've grown to fear and find repulsive in our bodies is a huge wake-up call. We can't continue to disregard this truth of life—that microbes are essential and we cannot live without them. It is a massive paradigm shift in the way we think. It calls into question the essence of who we are, and with that, our relationship not just *to* but *as an inextricable part of* the natural world. This, then, calls into question bigger concepts, such as our impact on the planet and on each other. It comes with an understanding that we as individuals and as a species are intimately connected to the earth, dirt, viruses, bacteria, and fungi—to everything! And everything is a part of us.

Realizing this not only creates an awareness of the inherent respect we should have toward each other and everything in nature, but opens us to the knowledge of the responsibility we have to walk lightly upon the earth. Our body is an expression of, and part of, Earth. As such, we would be well served to not only walk lightly and respect nature and others but recognize that we *are* nature. We are completely immersed in, made of, inseparable from, and affected by it. This reality is backed by new scientific data proving that everything from how we breathe, to what we eat, to where and how we live has an immediate impact on us, and specifically on the gut microbiome, as well as the microbiome in other places in or on the body.

Yes, that's right. There are microbial communities not just in the gut, but everywhere. You are not sterile; you couldn't survive if you were. There are microbes in internal organs, including in the uterine environment where a fetus grows, in every orifice, and all over the skin. You are literally an ecosystem. What's more, we don't just harbor these trillions of entities; we also emit them (as depicted in the illustration on the following page). Remember Pig-Pen from the Charlie Brown cartoons, with his permanent cloud of dust and bugs? That's you and me, and everything that is alive. We are all roaming around shedding our microbial dust clouds, leaving our imprint, literally, on every seat we temporarily inhabit. In doing so we leave a signature of microbial DNA as unique as a fingerprint. We exchange microbes with others in this way, even with our clothes on (researchers in one study even found vaginal bacteria unwittingly left behind on furniture by fully dressed women), and we also breathe them. This gives aura reading a whole new meaning!

In this book we will explore the nuts and bolts of the microbiome, both from the perspectives of modern science and Eastern medicine. We will examine what science actually knows, and what it doesn't know. We will look at what people are doing to manage and treat microbial imbalances, and whether those tactics are necessary or harmful. I will share everything you need to know about your microbiome and what you can do from a scientific standpoint to understand its health and

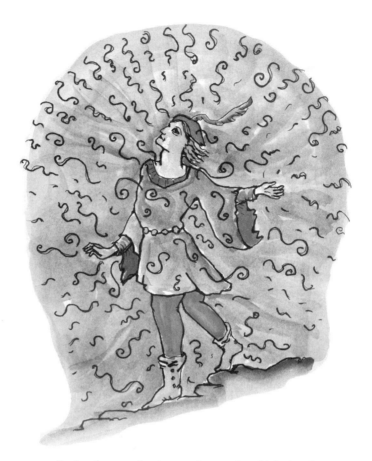

Each of us walks in a unique microbial cloud.

manage it. Interspersed within this discussion we will explore the microbiome from the perspective of Eastern medicine and practices, and how we can use those teachings to cultivate a healthier environment for the microbes in and on our bodies. That perspective was born from the ancient paradigm of holistic philosophy, which is thousands of years old and holds much wisdom about health and longevity.

Our current knowledge, research, and management of the microbiome is scarily limited. Modern scientists have barely begun to look to Eastern teachings, particularly those of India, China, and Tibet, to better inform and guide their hypotheses and research. Yet Eastern teachings are chock-full of detailed information explaining the importance of the gut; the role of digestion on the physical, mental, emotional, and spiritual health of the individual; and ways to manage gut health. The ancients knew how to diagnose and restore balance to a disordered gut flora; they just called it by other names. Very simply, the Chinese called it "spleen qi," and in India it was known as *agni*. The functions of these and other concepts in Eastern medicine relate in part to the function of the microbiome and its metabolites. Even lacking modern tools such as microscopes, Eastern medicine developed the concepts of microbes, pathogens, and pathogen types, and recognized qualities and activities they bring to the body that manifest as distinctive signs and symptoms that can be pathogen specific. Not only that, they developed sophisticated means to successfully treat disorders caused by these pathogens.

There are many instances where Western science has only in the past decade recognized structures in the human body that have been talked about by the Chinese for more than 2,000 years. Western scientists now recognize that these structures exist and have officially classified one as an organ, yet speculate as to the full purpose of its function. Chinese medicine doctors have known the newly recognized organs and structures in the body as well as the functions of the microbiome for millennia. For two of the newly recognized structures, they know not only their structure as in modern science, but also their function. They know how they work, what they're for, their role in health and disease, how diseases are stored in or travel through them, their relationships to the rest of the body, and how to treat their imbalances, or imbalances of other bodily tissues utilizing them.

In Chinese medicine, there is an organ in the body called the *san jiao,* or triple burner, or triple warmer. It is fascinating to anyone learning Chinese medicine, and is as responsible for the health of mind and body as any other major organ system. I believe one aspect of it, in addition to its correlation to the recently "discovered" interstitium (the fluid-filled spaces in between tissues), has to do with the microbiome and its metabolites. I also believe this microbial organ is connected with the fascia (connective tissue), circulatory system, cerebrospinal fluid, meninges, and lymphatic system, as a means to transport metabolites and for communication. From what I can gather, they all work together in one interconnected, vital fluid dance of balance.

Related to the san jiao in Chinese medicine is the *mo yuan*. Roughly this translates to "membrane source." Housed in the abdominal cavity and closely associated with the san jiao, this structure—which I equate to being the mesentery and omentum—was recognized as an organ by modern science in just the last few years. Scientists are now researching what it does and how, although Eastern medicine teachings already have some of that information. Again, it relates in part to the microbiome. This will be discussed more fully in chapter 4.

Similarly, Indian Ayurveda practitioners have known for millennia that most disease starts in the gut. Like their Chinese medicine peers, they have elaborate formulas for regulating gut health, and highly evolved yet simple dietary guidelines that anyone can follow to reestablish healthy digestive functioning. And if you think the digestive system doesn't take precedence over other bodily systems, imagine how you'd feel if you were looking forward to something but couldn't leave the house because you had diarrhea, or found yourself on a beach vacation with constipation, gas, and bloating the whole time. Then recognize that this is a daily reality for too many people.

Beyond discomfort and inconvenience, science has firmly established that some chronic, often debilitating diseases and cancers have in common certain bacterial communities in the gut, so we have more serious reasons to pay attention.

The homeostasis our microbiome constantly interfaces with the rest of the body to maintain has been emphasized by traditional cultures and medicine systems for thousands of years. Maintaining a balance of humors, *doshas* (types of mind-body structure and energy), elements, fluids, metabolic processes, thermoregulation, systems of circulation, bodily tissues, life airs, biological rhythms, and *yin* and *yang* is the crux of traditional preventive medicine, treatment, and vital longevity.

Ancient cultures had centenarians too: people who lived to 100 and beyond. They didn't have hand sanitizer and antibiotics, yet under normal and harsher circumstances than we experience in modern living, they still flourished and humanity survived. In such harsh circumstances without the comforts or conveniences of modern life, how did so many of them make it so long?

Researchers, explorers, travelers, and writers have been looking for a fountain of youth for millennia. They've looked under the microscope and in faraway places, hunted herbs, and delved into esoteric practices. They've encircled the globe in hopes of finding the "right" climactic or environmental conditions for human existence. Perhaps the wisdom to live with optimal health has been within us all along, and is as unique to each of us as our fingerprints.

That's right, your microbiome is as individual to you as your DNA, a snowflake in a storm, or your fingerprint. Just as there is only one you, there is only one combo of your individual microbiome. It is interesting to note that the aforementioned ancient medical systems also believed we have unique constitutional tendencies that require specific diet and lifestyle tweaks in order to stay balanced and, therefore, healthy. It is my belief that these ancient prescriptions for ultimate vitality and maximized good health are the best tools we have in lieu of enough science to know how to take optimal care of ourselves and our microbiomes. In other aspects of our lives we speak of the wisdom of the elders. We listen to our matriarchs and patriarchs and look to them for guidance in times of need and turmoil. Perhaps we ought to take this same approach to health and look to the foundational medicines of the East for guidance. They are vital, living systems of medicine in practice all over the world today.

Modern science repeatedly validates the teachings of these ancient medical traditions. What once were thought to be mystifying esoteric concepts are now coming to light as tangible aspects of physical reality. It is so interesting to learn from a modern scientific standpoint just how each of these things works. Take the circadian rhythm, or biological clock, for example. Three American scientists won a 2017 Nobel Prize for their discoveries about how biological rhythms govern human life, yet in Eastern medicine these rhythms have long been understood, and the lifestyle guidance specific to each individual's mind and body type laid out accordingly.

Likewise, Eastern medicines from both China and India have essential guidelines on how to use the sense of taste to regulate the body. In these traditions each organ is paired with a taste, and each taste activates or inactivates the subtle functions of the associated organs and tissues. Perhaps unsurprisingly, in the past few years scientists have also found bitter taste receptors normally present in the mouth that are widely expressed throughout the body, some in places we might not expect, such as the heart (more about this in chapter 2). And guess what: that correlates with what Eastern medicines have been teaching for millennia.

We now know the microbiome exists, how important it is, and that what it does has even more far-reaching influence over our quality of life than we ever dreamed possible before the last decade. Its maintenance and manipulation could have life-changing consequences for us. Since we don't currently have all the scientific data on it or how to utilize and maintain it, we can reference the time-tested wisdom of Eastern medicine for guidance. Although some of the terminology and concepts may be unfamiliar to us, they contain potential for great insight. I believe utilizing this knowledge can help each of us achieve our individual potential for the greatest health and quality of life possible. I see it happening in my clinic every single day. If properly understood and used as intended, Eastern medicine can be an invaluable resource to help us not only cope with and overcome mental fogginess, indigestion, fatigue, pain, and so on, but also maintain optimal well-being and profound vitality. And when Western science catches up to the successful practices of Eastern medicine, we will embrace that knowledge too.

Modern scientific research is limited by our current technology, so we can't possibly have all the answers to what makes the body work. It's possible that even smaller particles than the metabolites produced by our microbes will be revealed, or perhaps there is an energetic component to the living being that is yet to be "discovered." This is a perfect example of why we should not only respect the wisdom contained in Eastern medicines, but also seriously consider the wealth of information that comes from them.

There is a lot of information in this book, and there is a lot of information that isn't in this book. I want to make clear that this is neither a scientific paper nor pseudoscience. It is a delicately balanced blend of what the average intelligent, free-thinking, interested human being needs to know from both a modern scientific and medical perspective and the teachings of Eastern medicine, in order to understand the microbiome in a way that supports healing. I haven't gone into the cacophony of microbes and where they are and what they do; our knowledge of that is changing every day. What doesn't change are the guidelines Eastern medicine clearly lays out that we can follow to maintain optimal health.

We do have information on some key players, and those are included. You've probably already heard of *Lactobacillus,* for example, and its role in the gut and vaginal ecology. We know that *Prevotella* is associated with carbohydrate consumption (thus often dominant in vegans) and ferments dietary fiber into short chain fatty acids that may reduce inflammation. On the other hand, *Bacteroides*-dominant microbiomes, usually found in those eating diets high in animal products and low in fiber, are associated with increased secondary bile acid production, inflammation, and, as a result, higher risk of gastrointestinal disease. This classification of microbial dominant types, which Western science dubs "enterotypes," calls to mind the Ayurvedic concept of *vikruti,* or acquired constitution. Some of the microbes that colonize us sound scary, for example staph (*Staphylococcus*). It is common; we all have staph on and in us. It is only problematic when the system is somehow compromised and allows it to colonize out of control or take over a bodily tissue.

The terms *microbiome* and *microbiota* are often used interchangeably, but in this book I will use *microbiome* to address the entire mass of microbes in and on us, as well as their collective effects on the mind and body, unless I state specifically to which one I am referring, or it is implied by context. *Microbiota* refers to the entire collection of microbial communities that contribute to the composition of a human being, but I will veer away from this term for simplicity's sake. Other terms you will come across are *dysbiosis, symbiosis,* and *commensal. Dysbiosis* is an imbalance or malfunction in the microbiome of an individual. *Symbiosis* occurs when one or two organisms or groups living in close proximity benefit from one another. A *commensal* relationship is a long-term biological interaction in which one organism or species benefits while the other has a neutral reaction. These definitions as well as others related to the microbiome and Eastern medicine are also provided in the glossary at the back of the book for easy reference.

My interest lies largely in managing the microbiome holistically, using ancient science and wisdom as a guide, and implementing it into daily living. If you perceive the heavy influence of Eastern medicine as pseudoscience, go no further. If, however, you are serious about truly taking charge of your health and are open to living in greater accordance with natural cycles and by common sense in many cases, keep reading. If you're frustrated with feeling drowsy, bloated, unfocused, or unmotivated; or if your cycles are disrupted, your sleep disturbed, your emotions unpredictable or stuck in one gear, read on! The information contained in this book is for you. It weaves together what we have always known with what we are confirming daily by the scientific method. Why wait another century or more until all of Chinese medicine's or Ayurveda's principles are scientifically proven? Prove them in the lab of your own life by using Eastern wisdom to cultivate your microbiome now.

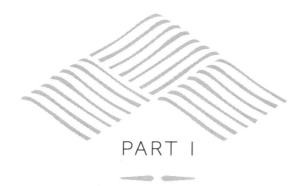

PART I

Modern Science Meets Ancient Wisdom

1
Everything but the Kitchen Sink

Exploring the Human Microbiome

For the first half of geological time our ancestors were bacteria.

RICHARD DAWKINS

Don't take this personally, but you are less than human. At least half of the genetic information that comprises your body and influences your mind—that which makes you feel most human—is actually not human. A substantial amount of your physical and genetic makeup, trillions of cells, are genetically "other." These other living, and in the case of viruses, nonliving entities are collectively and loosely known as the human microbiome. As mentioned earlier, this collective is so important and has so much impact on our health, longevity, and quality of life that it's often considered an organ in and of its own right. The little beings that comprise it include bacteria, fungi, and viruses, and we are only now, after hundreds of years of Western medicine and science, finally getting to know them. Our earliest glimpses into the microbial world started in the 1800s, but serious research didn't really kick into gear until about a decade ago.

The more we learn about this world, the more questions arise.

Fueling our curiosity is the hope that the information we glean will lead to the ability to cure diseases or alleviate their symptoms with manipulation of the microbiome. In fact, some scientists are coming to the conclusion that understanding the genetic material of our microbiome is as important as knowing all we can about the human genome. Below is a brief overview and introduction to some of what we currently do know, and some questions that arise as a result of our new knowledge.

We know our microbial inhabitants play a role in gene activation. They do not necessarily cause changes in the genetic material, but they can affect the way our genes express themselves, for better or for worse. They also affect estrogen levels in menstruating women. Maybe the gut microbiome plays a role in setting our biological clock. Maybe it causes menarche, or first menstruation, to begin, or perhaps an imbalance in the microbiome causes delayed onset. Could there be a community of metabolites specific to the microbes in the ovaries (which have microbiomes as well, and they may be different from left to right) and/or uterus we haven't discovered yet that is responsible for communicating this timing to the brain? Is it possible that sterilized, hormone-containing food in our diets creates a state of dysbiosis causing girls to start puberty prematurely? If that is the case, it may also play a role in male sexual development. It is conceivable because we know this happens elsewhere in nature. For example, there are sea creatures that don't mature into adults without a microbial-triggered gene activation.[1]

We know the gut microbiome communicates with the brain, and that it plays a major role in our ability to experience a sense of well-being. We also know it plays a role in the inflammatory response, and that an imbalance in the gut microbiome can cause anxiety and keep us in the stress response of fight-or-flight. We know a bit about the passing on of microbes to newborns: the amniotic fluid, the umbilical cord blood, and the placenta all contain microbial communities; the vaginal canal colonizes an infant born naturally; and babies born by C-section are colonized by the bacterial environment from the mother's abdominal skin and whatever is emitted by the delivering doctor or receiving nurse. Skin communities and vaginal communities are very different ecosystems. Studies show that C-section babies are more prone to obesity, asthma, and allergies later in life, so it seems probable there is a direct link between this statistic and skin colonization versus vaginal colonization.

In the case of various diseases, we know that specific communities are present in the guts of people with certain diagnoses, even if we don't yet know what manifested first: the disease or the imbalance in the microbiome. We've learned that when we treat people with certain gastrointestinal disorders by using healthy microbial communities from healthy people, the diseased state improves overall in the person with the imbalance. There is much more to learn, and it seems a new study is being published almost daily, but we already know for sure that the microbiome helps maintain our homeostasis, our vitality, and our overall well-being.

By far the most researched and talked about microbiome is that residing in the gastrointestinal (GI) tract, commonly known as "gut flora." It alone contains more than 3.3 million genes, contributing to and influencing our overall genetic makeup.[2] (We will explore the GI microbiome in the next chapter.) The microbiome incorporates all of the nonhuman cells/microbes/critters on and in the body. You may have had some of those little microbes today in yogurt, kimchee, a fermented beverage, or probiotic supplement.

There is also a *mycobiome,* or fungal microbiome, that we have less information about, but as is the case with the bacterial colonies we harbor, we are learning more about it every day. Some people take a probiotic supplement containing *Saccharomyces boulardii* in order to stop diarrhea associated with antibiotic use, or to crowd out an overgrowth of candida. There is also a high concentration of fungal helpers in the ear canal that are believed to keep the rest of the ear's microbial communities in check.[3]

In addition to the microbiome and mycobiome, our bodies also include a *virome.* The virome is a diverse collection of viruses that interact with the microbiome and affect us in ways we don't yet fully understand. Some sophisticated studies show these interactions may enhance or block infection, but the role viruses play in assisting our health has been little studied. Unfortunately, there are limitations to the technology available for this research.[4] Since we don't know much about the virome, and have little information about the mycobiome, we will focus on the best-researched aspect of the microbiome in this text, our beneficial bacteria.

The Skin You're In

There are microbiomes all over and in the human body. Let's start with the one on the largest organ: the skin. Living in follicles and glands as well as on the surface, the skin microbiome helps to protect against infection, and some scientists believe the microbial inhabitants on the skin may train killer T cells in their work of finding and destroying foreign, infected, or damaged cells.[5] This is aligned with the teaching in Chinese medicine that the skin contains a first line of defense in the immune system against potentially invading pathogens. This immunity in Chinese medicine is called *wei qi,* or defensive qi. Practitioners assess the functioning and quality of the defensive qi, and if it is deficient, can utilize acupuncture, diet, and herbal remedies to strengthen it. The skin microbiome has very similar friendly bacteria to the oral and gut microbiomes; they mostly differ in proportions particular to their classification by phylum.[6]

Not only is the skin colonized by microbes (bacteria, viruses, fungi), it is a home to mites as well. All of these players in the homeostasis of the skin make contributions to our good health in ways that our own human genome falls short.

The skin microbiome is affected by the environment, and studies have shown the presence of humidity and heat increases microbial counts on the back, armpits, and feet.[7] This makes sense from an Eastern medicine perspective. It is taught in Eastern medicine that like increases like, and that external environmental conditions influence the body's environment. It is also suspected that everything we apply to our skin affects the microbiome; it's just unclear exactly how at this time. We know that what we apply may alter the condition of the skin, so common sense speaks to the likelihood of microbial modification as a result. Are we feeding our good critters? Killing off the beings that live on us, regardless of their function? Altering the composition of colonies, and therefore altering their symbiotic effects on our health and well-being? This is food for thought the next time you reach for antibacterial soap or put some artificially fragranced lotion on your skin. What shampoo do you use? What lotion do you put on your face? Remember, in addition to being a protective barrier, the skin is a sponge. Much of what goes on it passes through it as well. Anyone who has had hormonal imbalances corrected by a tiny patch can attest to the power of absorbing something through the skin, as can those with skin sensitivities, such as a wool allergy. The skin breathes and interacts with its environment without our even knowing it.

Handwashing for Health

Maybe washing our hands to stay healthy works in ways we hadn't considered, not just by removing microbes so they don't enter through our nose, eyes, or mouth but ridding ourselves of microbes, or their metabolites, that otherwise might be absorbed through the skin or send messages to the gut and immune system through it.

The fact that the skin absorbs was known to the ancient Chinese and Indians, and is incorporated into a slew of treatments in both systems of medicine. In Eastern treatments, poultices, soaks, and topical treatments are the norm. They are advised for anything from nervous disorders to skin ailments, and from beauty treatments to traumatic injuries. I won't go over them in any detail here, as most are indicated for specific purposes according to diagnosis. What I can say is that in both Chinese medicine and Ayurveda, the skin is very important in both diagnosis and treatment. My guess is that one way poultices, soaks, and topical treatments work is to alter the microbiome in the area of focus, restoring homeostasis to the region—or to the region that correlates internally to that place on the body.

Most directly, researchers are finding a correlation between dysbiosis, or what is thought to be a pathological imbalance in the microbiome, internally and externally, and such skin issues as dermatitis, psoriasis, and eczema. In Eastern medicine, much can be told by the color, texture, temperature, sensitivity, laxity, density, markings, and moistness of the skin, as well as of the nails and hair.

Essential Oils, Friend or Foe?
Things to Consider before Using

We perceive substances called *oils* to be benign, as we use them regularly for cooking and nourishing our skin. In this more general sense of the word we are talking about bioavailable, unconcentrated oil. In contrast, *essential* oils are practically pharmaceutical-grade consolidations of plants and resins.

Essential oils are largely antimicrobial. As author and master herbalist David Crow points out, they are the distilled immune systems of plants. All the information that has come down through millennia to protect the plants is contained in each drop of oil. They have great potential for helping to keep us healthy when used in moderation in a balanced, well-informed manner. When overused, however, in addition to possibly triggering inflammatory reactions in the skin and respiratory systems, they may interfere with the beneficial microbes on the skin. These microbes knit together to form protective colony barriers against invaders, and excessive applications of essential oils have the potential to break those bonds. Additionally, some create photosensitivity and can result in bad burns if the skin is exposed to the sun. There is also the risk of irritating mucosal membranes if ingested. Essential oils are readily available but they are not all top quality, so think twice before ingesting them, and do so only at the behest of a qualified medical practitioner. I believe it is safest to use them selectively in a diffuser, occasionally in a carrier oil on the skin, or in small quantities in a steam inhalation to help clear the passages when the nose and sinuses are blocked.

Regional Differences

Each region of the skin has its own unique colonies in specific balance.

- **Navel.** There is a question as to what ways the microbiome of the navel influences our health overall. A 2012 study of the navel microbiome found 1,458 bacteria previously unknown to science. One person in the study harbored extreme microbes previously thought present only in thermal vents and ice caps. It is now thought that laparoscopic surgery through the navel may introduce these microbes to the body's interior.[8] Experts recommend regularly cleaning the navel with soap and water and gentle rubbing, but caution against alcohol as a cleanser, as it can disrupt the area's ecology.
- **Scalp.** A recent clinical study showed that an imbalance in the bacterial community of the scalp may be implicated in the production of dandruff.[9]
- **Armpits and Genitals.** I'm sure you can imagine how the communities on and around the armpits and genitals must be different from those on the forearm or face. The way these microbial communities utilize our bodily secretions is what causes each of our distinct odors.

Researchers have found that in the armpits of study participants, people who don't use deodorant or antiperspirant had more than double the population of *Corynebacterium*. This microbe works with the body to maintain or restore balance, and is present in the vagina, fighting off pathogens. The study leaders divided participants into three groups: Some wore only antiperspirant, then stopped after several days; some wore deodorant, then stopped; and some wore neither. After stopping the study, the deodorant- and antiperspirant-users had triple the staph microbes compared to non-users, and the fewest corynebacteria, the ones known to provide a strong defense against pathogens.[10] They also exhibited the greatest diversity of microbes, which may be linked to better health in the gut, but is not necessarily so for the armpit.

Healthy armpits contain an enormous number of bacteria but not a great variety, according to scientist Chris Callewaert, an expert on armpit (axilla) microbes. In fact, a greater diversity of microbes in the armpits usually equates to worse body odor because increased diversity in this area usually means more diverse colonies of bad bacteria—the ones that produce a foul smell. Dr. Callewaert has been working with transplanting armpit microbial communities in order to address bad body odor. He's found that people who are more genetically similar have greater success rates with the procedure, so he uses family members in his experiments.[11] In preparation for the transplant, the armpits of the malodorous recipient are sterilized, while the sweeter-smelling donor is encouraged to let bacteria flourish. Then the donor microbe community is applied to the recipient's armpits, which can't be washed for a week. Dr. Callewaert reports semi-permanent to permanent results.[12]

Research from the University of York shows that staph is making the biggest contribution to foul underarm odor.[13] A National Public Radio article describing the findings states, "Most deodorants [and antiperspirants] block sweat glands or kill off underarm bacteria. Blocking the sweat glands sometimes leads to irritated or swollen skin. And given all the new research into the complexity of the human microbiome, the researchers are a little anxious that deodorants may kill good bacteria, too."[14] They aren't sure we should be killing any bacteria, as it can upset the balance, potentially allowing for the stink-causing staph and other potentially harmful species to run rampant. Instead, researchers are looking for ways to add friendly bacteria to the armpits that hopefully will colonize and take up more space and air than their stink-causing counterparts, crowding them out.

More research is needed to understand how the skin microbiome plays a role in various skin diseases, as well as how to encourage the dominance of helpful players and mitigate the offenders.

The Mouth

The mouth is called the gateway to the stomach in Eastern medicine, and it is the gatekeeper for potentially trillions of microbes entering the body—thousands per swallow.[15] The mouth microbiome's composition overlaps that of the colon's by about 45 percent![16] Some researchers posit that what we eat affects our teeth less directly than it affects the healthy balance of mouth microbes. They believe that it isn't sugar, for example, directly causing cavities, but the dysbiosis, or disruption to the healthy balance of the microbial communities in the mouth caused by sugar consumption that is the culprit.

There is increasing evidence in support of a direct connection between mouth health and systemic health. Basically, what is happening in the mouth is a reflection of what is going on in the rest of the body. This may also mean that what is happening in the mouth has a role to play in *causing* what's happening in the rest of the body. Here we can again refer to Eastern medicine, which has the detailed evaluation tool of tongue diagnosis, which is tremendously limited in Western medicine. Tongue diagnosis is just what it sounds like: looking at the tongue to determine the state of the insides of the body and the functioning of the mind. The tongue's coating, shape, and color reflect the quality of digestion and metabolism, the presence of toxins, and the state of the microbiome.

In addition, Eastern medicine hygiene techniques such as tongue scraping and oil pulling, or *kavala,* are being used more regularly now in the West with promising results. Although we don't have much trial data, coconut oil, for example, contains vitamin E (an antioxidant) and has antibacterial and anti-fungal properties, as does sesame oil, which is traditionally recommended for oil pulling. Unlike many mainstream mouthwashes containing alcohol, which may contribute to dysbiosis, using oil may actually be nourishing to the friendly bacteria in the mouth. Beyond the oil's potentially nourishing and antimicrobial properties, there may be something to how the oil's viscosity changes during the pulling process, in addition to the sucking and swishing, that accounts for its numerous beneficial effects.

Many of us have heard the term *leaky gut.* The mouth may also have increased permeability of the membranes that allows pathogenic microbes to migrate into systemic circulation. This means leaky gut doesn't just happen in the gut, but can happen across other membranes as well. This is just one way the mouth may affect the rest of the body, potentially leading to increased inflammation. Eastern medicine recognizes that disturbed physiological factors can come from pretty much anywhere and migrate to places in the body where they don't belong, wreaking havoc.

In a recent interview for the blog *Ask the Dentist,* ethnopharmacologist Cass Nelson-Dooley answers a question about the connection between periodontal disease and inflammatory bowel disease. She states, "A mouth that is sick is seeding the entire GI tract with bad bugs every day."[17] This may be hugely problematic, especially if the beneficial microbes in the gut are not diverse enough or the gut is overrun with microbes that are creating imbalance in the system. Steven Lin, D.D.S., writes, "Probiotic strains of bacteria are known to perform protective functions in the mouth. For example, some strains release acids that keep the harmful bacteria that cause tooth decay under control. Others protect against strains that cause gum disease and bad breath."[18]

So how do we maintain a good mouth environment? Eating a good diet is key, as is reducing or eliminating broad-spectrum mouthwashes that annihilate good bacteria as well as bad. In addition to oil pulling, if it isn't contraindicated for your current presentation (which may include head or neck, including mouth, pathologies), maintaining consistency with tongue scraping, flossing, and brushing is, of course, critical. Breathing through your nostrils rather than your mouth is also beneficial for oral microbiome health. Breathing through the mouth may dry out the mucosa and contribute to dysbiosis.

A study released in January 2019 suggests a strong link between the bacteria *Porphyromonas gingivalis,* the bug that stimulates gingivitis—and Alzheimer's disease. Not only is there a link, the study claims this microbe is a primary causative factor, being intimately tied to the amyloid plaques present in the brains of many Alzheimer's patients. By-products of the microbe's activity, called gingipains, were found in the majority of brains tested of people who died from the disease. As part of the study researchers infected mice orally with *Porphyromonas gingivalis,* then administered a gingipain inhibitor. It was found that the inhibitor was more effective at curing the mice of their gingivitis than the commonly administered antibiotic prescribed to humans.[19] Although more research is needed, including human trials for the gingi-pain inhibitor, this is yet another example of the link between a member of the microbial community and its impact on health or disease, both locally and in other parts of the body.

The Nose Knows

Within the nose there are very interesting and unexpected factors at play. We know that the nasal passages are lined with hairs that help filter potentially harmful entities and substances from entering deeper into the body, but did you know they also have ridges that affect your mood? The nose contains turbinates that swirl and shape the flow of air entering the body, and affect how it hits the back of the cavity, influencing the brain. This flow, if strong enough and nurtured with healthy breathing, can affect the limbic system and alter our mood. It may be that the microbes lining the nasal passages have a role to play in changing the shape of this landscape. In classical yoga, nose breathing is so important that there is a comprehensive system of breathing practices called *swara* that deals with different ways to regulate air flow through the nostrils. It helps to induce meditative and other mental states, and helps practitioners to identify and align with their biological clocks and other cycles of nature.

It is optimal to breathe through the nose instead of the mouth. This is not only good for the microbial communities helping to keep your mouth healthy, but also good practice for keeping your lungs healthy. Think about how dryness affects you when forced hot air is first turned back on during the winter. It wreaks havoc with people's mucosal membranes. When the wetness dries, filtering is decreased and pathogens can more easily enter the deeper areas of the respiratory pathways. Additionally the dryness can affect the throat, cause coughing, and be just plain uncomfortable. It is therefore recommended to make a habit out of breathing in and out through the nose at all times of year. Breathing in through the nostrils, instead of the mouth, filters pathogens, dust, and other irritants. Exhaling through the nose allows the balmy, moist air from the lungs to rewarm and remoisten the nasal passages. What an ingenious, simple mechanism for self-regulation! Nature is incredibly efficient. This is the temperate, humid environment we want to cultivate for our nasal, sinus, bronchi, and lung mucusa and for our friendly microbes.

There is literally a bittersweet battle raging in your nose right now between bacteria that are working to keep each other in check. Different strains in the nasal cavity help to keep you healthy by secreting amino acids that activate taste receptors on your cells and prevent things like sinusitis from developing. Molecules on, or secreted by, bacteria can activate bitter taste receptors in the sinuses that produce antimicrobial molecules. Other bacteria directly or indirectly activate sweet receptors that produce further balancing results.[20]

Yes, you did just read that we have taste receptors on cells in our sinuses. As mentioned earlier, we have taste receptors on cells in lots of places in our bodies that are far removed from the tongue. In Eastern medicine, foods and medicines are classified by taste in order to intentionally alter, activate, or deactivate biological processes. One simple example of this is in using bitter medicinals to clear heat (inflammation) from the body. As explained above, this is exactly what is happening in the head naturally, via the microbiome, without our interference.

Eastern teachings specify which foods should be eaten for which internal environment or individual constitution at any given time of the year according to taste and thermogenic properties. In Western science there is less recognition, understanding, or even awareness of the influence of taste on our physiology. We tend to see food according to calories, macromolecules, and nutritive constituents. This is one of the reasons I encourage people to steer toward a diet that is steeped in Eastern wisdom. I see many diet plans and cookbooks that encourage eating for the microbiome but fall short of what we can be doing to optimize one's microbiome as an individual. They do not take into account the digestibility of the food, the way the food is combined, how it is eaten, the season in which it is eaten, or the individual's body type.

Microbiology has recognized that the tastes sweet and bitter carry out specific tasks in the nasal and sinus cavities. There are two theories that may help to explain it:

1. Sweet secretions protect what we may think of as symbiotic and commensal (good) microbial communities. More unfavorable microbes eat the glucose that causes the sweet taste. This then activates bitter taste receptors on cells that turn on antimicrobial secretions, keeping the bad guys and gals in check.*

2. Sweet compounds (not glucose), like certain amino acids that are produced by some bacteria, may be suppressive to the antimicrobial secretions, which actually allows the commensal (good) guys to fully colonize.[21]

---

*For the record, the microbes that make up the microbiome in or on any part of the body are not generally lumped into good and bad categories, this is merely for explanation of this concept. *Dysbiosis* does not necessarily mean bad microbes, it means that the ecosystem in an area of the body is out of whack.

Scientists are studying how to better understand this phenomena so that they may utilize taste in the nose to help treat people suffering with chronic sinusitis.

Tricky Tonsils

The tonsils play an active role in immunity. Seated at the junction of the oro- and nasopharynx are three sets of them: the adenoids, palatine tonsils, and lingual tonsils. This lymphatic/epithelial tissue is most popular for being removed in childhood, when it may become chronically inflamed and swell, leading to breathing difficulty. We may as a culture view them as disposable, but the tonsils filter and trap incoming pathogens from the mouth and nose. They also notify the immune system of the presence of a potential pathogen so the rest of the body can initiate preventive measures to stop their spread and catch them if they make a break. There are resident communities of friendly microbes in this area as well, and their balance may be key to preventing chronic tonsillitis.

Eye of the Beholder

The eyes also have a unique microbiome. A study done on mice and published in the journal *Immunity* shows commensal bacteria resident to the ocular surface, which keep the eyes free from infection. Researchers found that these microbes work by stimulating the production of interleukin, an immune-signaling protein. This is produced by mucosal immune cells, and its presence attracts white blood cells to an area to boost immunity. In this case the area is the cornea.[22] Once again, as in the nose, the microbes living in and around us work with our human cells like a team to help keep us healthy.

In Eastern medicine the eyes are the window to the soul. The vibrance and vitality the eyes exude reflect the *shen,* or spirit, the state of mental and emotional health of the individual.

Vagina Chronicles

Let's move more deeply into the body now and explore what we know about the internal microbiomes. The vagina hosts a complex microbiome of bacteria, viruses, and fungi. In this environment, diversity is key. The job of the primary bacterial colonizer in the vaginal canal, *Lactobacillus,* is to interact with the host's own cells to keep mucus production in balance and protect from invaders.[23] This creates an acidic environment that helps protect against things like sexually transmitted infections, bacterial vaginosis, and pelvic inflammatory disease. It also helps guard against the overgrowth of potentially harmful bacteria, viruses, and yeasts that might otherwise become too abundant.[24]

Although research is needed, it is now known that pretty much everything can disturb the vaginal microbiome's balance, including menstruation. Things as seemingly unrelated to this area of the body as what goes into our mouths can adversely affect our vaginal microbial balance. Antibiotics are notorious for wiping out *Lactobacillus.* Any woman who has taken a course of antibiotics and ended up with a vaginal yeast infection knows very well just how related it all is. Decreasing the numbers of certain lactobacilli allows other critters—in this case, candida—to thrive. Hormonal contraceptives and excessive alcohol consumption also affect the vaginal microbiome, as do diet and aging. I think it makes sense, given all the science available, that any birth control affects the vaginal microbiome, even those that aren't believed to create systemic reactions. Anything that enters the vagina may change its microbial composition. That includes substances from sexual activity, like semen and lubricants. For this reason, it is generally recommended to avoid douching.[25]

Once the microbial composition of the vaginal canal is compromised, undesirable entities can enter into even deeper places—the uterus, fallopian tubes, and ovaries. There is some evidence that vaginal dysbiosis, or a resulting infection, can even affect a woman's fertility, or if she does get pregnant, the fetus.[26] Some reports cite the presence of adverse bacteria in the uterus causing recurrent miscarriage.

Recurrent Miscarriage in Chinese Medicine

In Chinese medicine, many female fertility issues and recurrent mis-carriages are considered the result of patterns that may be correct-able with bodywork modalities, including acupuncture, and medicinal preparations (herbal formulas). Instead of addressing the issue as a defect of the woman's hormonal or immune system, Chinese medi-cine sees it as the result of an imbalance in the woman's constitu-tional factors and internal environment, which may be associated with complications from one of several pathogenic influences such as excess heat, cold, dampness, phlegm, or dryness. This imbalance may be caused by or result in fluid or vitality circulation issues or one or more of these pathogenic influences being lodged in the uterus. Such an influence might be classified by modern science as the result of unchecked microbial agents entering the upper reproductive tract.

Research indicates there is indeed a placental microbiome, an area that, up until recently, was believed to be sterile. In addition, some experts believe the placenta can be contaminated by microbes that may affect the growth and development of the fetus, and potentially lead to preterm labor and delivery.[27] Much more research needs to be done, as we don't currently know what the role of the mother's microbiome is in fetal development, let alone what the composition of a healthy, life-supporting womb environment should be.

In the Womb and Beyond

As we noted earlier, there is a marked difference in the microbiomes of newborns born vaginally and those born by Cesarean section. Those born without intervention are colonized by the mother's vaginal micro-biome through the mouth, face, and bodily exposure. Babies born via C-section are largely colonized, at least initially, by microbial entities from the mother's skin. Any attending delivery personnel who come into contact with the infant may also transfer microbes. C-section babies are shown to be more prone to developing allergies and asthma, and there is speculation that it might be due to having skin and gut microbiomes that largely resemble the mother's skin versus her vagina. Because of this, some people are now swabbing the vaginal canal of C-section mothers and administering a smear of beneficial colonies to the newborn's mouth, face, and body. In one experiment, those born by C-section and inoculated after birth with their mother's vaginal microbiome were shown after one month to have a gut microbiome that more resembled the mother's vagina.[28]

There is strong evidence that even before a baby is born it is being programmed by the mother's microbiome, and that the mother's microbial metabolites influence the brain development of her fetus.[29] A researcher at the University of Michigan who studies fMRI scans of babies has observed that the amygdala's connections to the rest of the brain structures are stronger in those with a less diverse microbial gut composition.[30] The amygdala is the primitive part of the brain that gets activated to respond to strong emotional states, such as fear and anger. This finding may indicate that the microbiome has a strong influence on how a baby develops its personality, and perhaps whether it is more prone to experience strong emotions, such as fear and anger.[31]

The Bladder

The bladder was formerly believed to be sterile, but now we know that it too has a microbiome, and that there is a distinct connection between the urinary and vaginal microbiomes. The bladder microbiome is influenced by diet and lifestyle factors, and altered by urinary tract disease. It is also associated with urinary incontinence in women. Researchers are hopeful that further exploration of the urinary tract microbiome will create treatment options other than antibiotics for women with recurrent urinary tract infections.[32] Studies are currently underway in hopes of discovering whether or not the urinary microbiome also has a role to play in bladder cancer.

Testes

Researchers have found that healthy testes are home to a diversity of microbes from four major families. Like the bladder, the testes were previously believed to be a sterile environment, but access to new technologies has now given scientists the tools to "discover" these diverse microbial inhabitants. They do so by tracking them through their DNA.[33]

There is evidence that an imbalance in the testes microbiome may play a significant role not only in some male fertility issues, but also in production of sperm. Men with a certain condition that doesn't allow sperm to exit the body with the semen were found to have decreased microbial diversity. Further, men who produced no sperm had only one group of microbes present.[34] This makes me think of how Eastern traditions prescribe moderation in sexual activity, particularly for men, as it is believed that overindulgence can weaken the essence. Perhaps this is because too much sexual activity damages microbial diversity. Western researchers also think there may be a link between microbiomes in other places in the body and prostate issues, but more studies are needed.

The Lungs

Another site in the body previously believed to be sterile is the lung environment. Forgive me for being critical here, but why would we think anything in the body is sterile? It seems a childish notion. There is hardly a place on Earth, if any, that is not inhabited by microbes. Even the most extreme environments harbor thriving resident communities. All creatures have mites and bugs on them and in them. We are no different.

The ecosystem in the lungs is particularly fascinating because it changes with every breath. Having a background in yoga, and a particular interest in the mental, emotional, psychospiritual, and physical dynamics of the breath, I find this realm very interesting. Unlike the other microbiomes, including the one in the gut when it's healthy, the lungs have a bidirectional means of transporting and exchanging microbes. This means that instead of one primary direction of movement (as in the case of the GI tract where microbes travel from the mouth, in one direction, to the anus), the lungs bring in *and* send out. The respiratory pathway has two entrances that also serve as exits. As a serious student of the breath, I know that we have immense influence over our respiratory health, that we can alter it consciously, and that the quality of our respiration has a direct effect on our physical, mental, and emotional well-being. It follows that it may also directly influence the quality and/or activity of the microbiome both in the lungs and the gut.

In an article citing a study done of the lung microbiome in 2017, Robert P. Dickson, M.D., states, "The lungs are our largest interface with the outside environment, with 70 square meters of surface area. That's thirty times the size of the skin and twice the size of the gastrointestinal tract."[35] As it turns out, the lung microbiome most closely resembles that of the mouth. Researchers believe this happens largely as a result of microaspiration, or the inhalation of microbes into the upper reaches of the lungs. There are mechanisms in place that don't allow much to enter, and it seems that what does get in also exits. Although some microbes do inhabit the deeper air sacs, called "alveoli," researchers think the lung microbiome is largely a transient community kept in check by both the host's immune system and the ability to expel the microbes via coughing and ciliary action. It's when the immune system is weakened for some reason, or microbial inhabitants overstay their welcome, that the microbiome becomes dysbiotic and causes infection or disease.[36] I think researchers are likely to discover that the lung microbiome is comprised of more residents than they currently believe. Curiously, the lungs of some critically ill patients contain the microbial inhabitants of the gut, which indicates the importance of strong immunity.[37] It also suggests that there may be a mode of travel from the gut to the lungs for these microbes. From an Eastern medicine perspective these communities of microbes would travel via the circulation, fluid pathways, meridians, and san jiao.

Interesting factoids about the lung microbiome are that the ratio of bacterial to human cells in the lungs is 100 microbial cells to every 1000 host cells.[38] Another is that we are subject to microbial lung colonization from birth. There is a shift in the microbial composition of the lungs in the infant over the first two weeks of life toward microbes that encourage resistance to allergens. These data suggest acquisition of a lung microbiome is an important early-life event necessary to protect the lung from injurious responses to inhaled antigens.[39] I wonder just how early. There have been findings of microbes in the placenta, but more research is needed to understand their function: Are they alive? How do they get there? Do they influence the immune system or other development of the fetus?[40] This also makes me wonder if the proteins secreted by the fetus that initiate labor could be triggered by microbial activity.

In researching the lungs, I was unable to find any reputable studies on the effects of intentional breathing techniques or of healthy breathing on the lung microbiome. If I had, it would be covered here in depth. It is interesting to me that a natural, healthy breath involves inhaling and exhaling through the nose, and that unconsciously breathing through the mouth on a regular basis is considered pathological. In addition to not allowing for optimal filtration of particles while mouth breathing, it may also be that mouth breathing allows for a greater number of microbes, more than would be inspired through nasal breathing, to enter the lungs. It makes sense that if this is the case, it would force the body to work harder to keep the communities in manageable numbers, overworking the immunity in this area and making it more difficult to stay healthy. In addition, mouth breathing is more likely to dry the mucosa that comes in contact with the inhaled air and in that way also affect microbial activity of the lungs and homeostasis.

The breathing exercises in yoga practices, categorized as *kriyas* (cleansing actions) and *pranayama* (vitality control), serve various purposes that benefit the health of the entire body-mind complex. There are specific exercises that assist one in releasing some of the older dead air in the bottom of the lungs and stale energy from the lungs in general that may be of great benefit to those who have issues with the cough reflex or ciliary action. These techniques may also increase gas exchange with pulmonary capillaries and prevent the development of additional dead space in the lungs. They may be just what the average, healthy person needs to keep ahead of pathogens in the winter months, or allergens at any time of year. Some of these exercises will be elaborated on in chapter 7.

Neti (nasal cleansing) pots are widely popular and are used quite extensively in the American yoga community. Although there are now variations on the shape and materials, a neti pot is a small container with a nasal spout that is used to flush salinated water through the nose via the nostrils, in order to filter out particles and mucus that may be stuck in the sinus cavity. When I was studying in India, two teachers from the same lineage, the one most American yoga practitioners are influenced by, cautioned against the use of neti pots. These teachers insisted that the saline, especially when neti pots are used regularly, gets into the lungs and can cause disease. Perhaps this is because the saline water is microaspirated and creates an imbalance in the lung tissue or its microbiome. If you do use a neti pot, it is recommended only to use sterile water. This caution comes after incidences made the news of pathogenic amoebas, believed to be transmitted to the brains of two people through the tap water in their neti pots, resulted in those people's untimely deaths. I'm not advising against the use of neti pots, but I wouldn't recommend trying it for the first time when you are sick, and I recommend moderation in usage.

Researchers suspect that the lung microbiome plays a primary role in our overall immunity and homeostasis. Maybe healthy humans harbor lung microbiomes not just because microbes are accidentally aspirated and our immunity is keeping them in check, but because they are helping to keep us healthy and alive. We know the diversity of symbiotic microbial communities is minimized in diseased lungs. Our scientific knowledge of connections among these microbes, their metabolites, gases in the respiratory tract, and our immune and other cells is grossly lacking. It is my sense that this ecosystem is just as important as the one in the gut or elsewhere in or on the body.

It has been my intention with this chapter to give you a substantial introduction to and understanding of some of the body's microbiomes. By no means could everything be covered in this chapter, but I hope I've given you enough to be in awe of the microbiome and how it works. If I've left an area untouched in this chapter, keep in mind that this is merely an overview, and we will revisit some of these areas later in the book when exploring how Eastern medicine treats the microbiome holistically. I hope this has opened your eyes to the extent of the microbiomes of your body, and the importance of their balance in your good health. Next we will turn to the gastrointestinal microbiome, which gets its own chapter since it is the one we know the most about, including how it is connected to and influences the body, brain, and mind.

2

The Kitchen Sink

Digestion and the
Gastrointestinal Microbiome

All disease begins in the gut.
HIPPOCRATES

"Mommy, eating food is magic!" my daughter announced. How is that? "Because I put the food in my mouth and it goes down into my stomach, but my body is closed. How does it go in when I am closed? It's because of magic." I have to say my child's explanation of how digestion works was one of the cutest things I've heard. And she's right: in some ways, it is magic, not just because the human body is a wonder, but because modern science still has much to learn about just how it functions. Western science still doesn't know all the hormones in the body or the extent to which they direct us. Look at all the diseases we have yet to find cures for or prevent! And then there is the microbiome.

Modern science is just at the tip of the iceberg when it comes to understanding the microbiome and all of its functions. It seems the more we explore, the more interesting information we glean, and the more questions surface and prompt the need for further studies. I've already mentioned some of the ways the microbiome operates and where we know it exists in and on us. Now let's delve into the depths of the gastrointestinal tube.

My daughter said her body is closed. To a three-year-old child, that may seem the case. In actuality, the alimentary canal, or gastrointestinal (GI) tract, is open to the outside world at both ends: the mouth and the anus. The GI tract, or gut, includes the mouth, esophagus, stomach, and small and large intestines. The digestive system as a whole integrates the function of many other accessory organs, including the tongue, teeth, salivary glands, liver, pancreas, gallbladder, and digestive glands. To fully understand digestion requires knowledge of all of these tissues and organs and how they interact. For the purposes of this chapter and exploring the gut microbiome in general, we are focusing only on the GI tract.

When we chew, the teeth break down food, and salivary glands in the mouth secrete enzymes that start breaking down starches. The tongue mashes it all around, mixing the salivary juices with the chewed food, then pushes it back to be swallowed. The microbiome in the mouth monitors what is going in to the deeper regions of the body. Down food goes, through the esophagus to the stomach. The stomach lining is highly acidic, allowing for the further breakdown of food and the annihilation of incoming microbes. It sloshes the food around in the acid, and then empties it into the small intestine.

The small intestine is where water, bile, and enzymes mix with food and turn it into something unrecognizable. The small intestine draws in water from the bloodstream to help break down the food and pushes it back and forth, making sure it all gets exposed to its vast surface area. This area is enormous thanks to the help of intestinal villi. These are little fingerlike projections that line the tract here and increase its surface area allowing for greater nutrient absorption. The gallbladder adds bile from the liver, and this mixes with the digestive enzymes of the pancreas.

The food is then pushed into the large intestine, where nutrients are produced and absorbed, as is water—anywhere from a cup and a half to a quart a day. Imagine how precise that filtration system needs to be!

In general, the GI tract is made up of four layers of tissue: the mucosa, submucosa, muscularis externa, and serosa. The mucosa contains mucus-secreting cells and is where the microbiome lives. In addition to mucus, the mucosa produces digestive enzymes (many manufactured by the microbes here), and hormones. The mucosa absorbs the final products of digestive breakdown, our nutrients, and helps protect against pathogens. The mucus it secretes protects our insides against the enzymes digesting our food. It also acts as a barrier stopping unwanted microbes and debris from getting through to deeper tissues.

Surrounding the mucosa is a layer of connective tissue that contains lymph tissue and nerve fibers known as the submucosa. It has as many lymph vessels as there are capillaries. The lymph helps to trap pathogens, while the capillaries absorb nutrients. After this comes the muscularis externa, responsible for peristalsis, or the moving of food through the GI tract, as well as forming the sphincters that control the passage of food from one part of the gut to another.[1] Proper coordination of the nerves and muscles here is imperative for healthy movement in the GI tract. This constant movement is useful for moving not only food through, but transient pathogens, helping to prevent them from adhering. Lastly, we have the serosa, or visceral peritoneum.[2] This lining is continuous with the tissue lining the entire abdominal cavity and its organs, known as the mesentery. The mesentery, recently given organ status, is a thoroughfare of blood vessels, lymphatics, and nerves that provide circulation, immunity, and ultimately connection among all the internal structures it encompasses. It suspends and anchors the internal organs and stores fat. We will discuss the mesentery in more detail in chapter 4.

To reiterate, the digestive process begins in the mouth. When we eat food, the salivary glands kick into action and begin secreting saliva—basically blood without the red blood cells—in order to break down the sugars it contains, and we increase the surface area by chewing. Eastern medicine, however, goes beyond this description. Eastern medicine recognizes that the quality of digestion begins in the mind.

The Mind's Role in Digestion

If we're upset, angry, or anxious, it can have an adverse effect on the quality and quantity of digestive juices, enzymes, and peristalsis, and we are likely to experience a range of signs and symptoms including brain fog, fatigue after eating, mucus congestion, abdominal pain, bloating, gas, constipation, loose bowel movements, and acid reflux.

Some people avoid food when they're upset but some turn to food, probably in an attempt to soothe themselves, because chewing and eating have a calming effect on the mind and body. Chemicals that get activated or released during the process of digestion can also be soothing, as they have proven antidepressant and pain-relieving effects. As an aside, I think that for some people the mechanism behind self-soothing with food plays a role in jaw clenching and grinding, and ultimately in temporomandibular joint disorders (TMJD). It could be that in the absence of food, the mentally soothing action of chewing manifests as clenching or grinding.

Those who suffer from lack of appetite when upset are probably better off in the short term because they aren't ingesting food they don't need at a time when their digestion might be subpar. The problem is that if the upset is chronic, they aren't being truly nourished. When the body isn't being nourished, it changes the microbial balance in the gut, affecting the mind adversely and creating more angst. Like eating to self-soothe, this could be a contributing factor to eating disorders, which are a massive problem in our culture.

I am cautious about what dietary recommendations I give to people if I suspect they have an unhealthy relationship with food, and usually focus on balancing their nervous system, their breath, and their mind. I encourage them to focus on the mind because the trapped mental and emotional energy related to eating or not is also problematic for digestion. The energetic of the control and holding that is created by food fixation is not good for the gut. It is a form of tension that's held in the mind and body and is just as detrimental as any other pattern of constraint. So often constraint, stagnation, holding, and grasping are at the root of the imbalance I see manifesting as many different ailments. Few of these are generated by what the body is being fed, but by the mind and how it is affecting and being reflected in the body.

This is why I say digestion, from a holistic, Eastern-medicine perspective, begins with the mind. The result is, of course, also physical. Chronically withheld food leads to changes in the metabolism that can lead to weight issues and inflammation. In Eastern medicine we say the agni (digestive juices) will burn the *kapha* (mucosa) for food, or that fire can consume the yin. In other words, the body will eat itself if not properly fed. There are many factors that go into what happens on a diet or a fast, one possibility being that some of the microbes inside you may start to starve and begin eating the mucus layer of the digestive tract because they need a food source. They, too, are trying to survive. This is also their world, and they'll eat anything that can be food for them to stay alive, just as a human would.

Eastern medicine holds that not eating regularly or in a balanced fashion weakens the immune system. The spleen qi, or the metabolism, is responsible for providing nutrition to keep the wei qi, or immune system, in good working order. Without adequate provisions, the immune cells cannot have sufficient numbers, communication breaks down among various parts of the body, and a multitude of ills may result, such as inflammatory problems, or pathogens sneaking in and potentially hiding out to reemerge at a later time.

In terms of overeating, the body can take only so much. If you're upset, and the acids, bile, enzymes, and movement get out of balance with one another, or the quality of the juices isn't optimal, eventually you may have undigested foodstuff in the GI tract. Eastern medicine considers this undigested foodstuff to be a primary player in leaky gut, as it is an irritant. In leaky gut, for one reason or another the protective mucosal layer doesn't trap what it's supposed to, and/or gaps form between epithelial cells lining the intestines. This causes the gut-associated lymphoid tissue (GALT) to go into high alert. The integrity

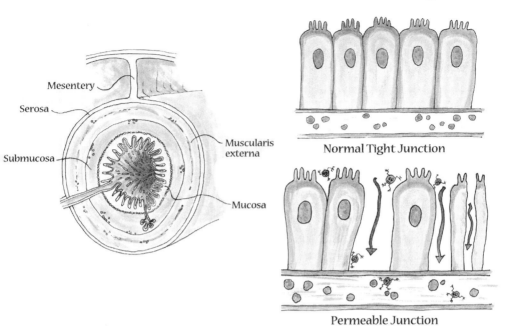

An intestinal cross section shows the layers of tissue in the GI tract. The image on the right illustrates the gap junctions between epithelial cells as they are ideally (top), and then when they become compromised (bottom), which leads to increased permeability.

of the gut lining is imperative. The fact that 70 percent of our immune cells reside in the gut is a testament to this.[3] The intestinal cells absorb nutrients for nourishment and distribution to the rest of the body, and also pull toxins from the blood for elimination.[4]

The Truth about Toxins

There are many types of toxins—from environmental toxins, to by-products of cellular metabolism stuck in the distal tissues, to mental and emotional toxins. The ancients were aware that the body has built-in detoxification mechanisms and devised protocols to support them. Ayurvedic medicine uses an intricate cleansing regimen called *panchakarma* that rounds up toxins, called *ama,* and guides them largely to the digestive tract, where practitioners use oils, herbs, and exercises to make sure they are released from the body. Chinese medicine describes dampness, phlegm, phlegm damp, heat, phlegm heat, wind, and cold as pathogenic factors that must be eliminated or transformed, oftentimes through various herbal remedies, purgation therapies, emesis (vomiting), and diaphoresis (profuse perspiration).

Author Alejandro Junger, M.D., states in his book *Clean Gut,* that "the gut's good bacteria neutralize about 40 percent of the toxins we consume in our food, acting as a kind of satellite liver."[5] This statement blew me away. If the microflora in the gut are not diverse and the beneficial ones well-fed; communicating well among themselves and with the immune system, the brain, and the rest of us; or if their environment is not conducive to their optimal functioning, then either the liver has to work harder or we become more toxic. This toxicity that is generated in the gut can overwhelm the body's innate defenses and create inflammation and disease. In Eastern medicine we classify this detox mechanism of the gut microbiome as an aspect of agni (digestive fire) and the functioning of the spleen qi (the power to transform). If the agni is damaged or the spleen qi deficient, we simply cannot process substances properly or thoroughly eliminate toxins.

The lymph tissue surrounding the gut sends immune cells back and forth into the intestines. When it does, it's checking for what gets a pass, or what needs to be stopped in its tracks or tagged as nonself. When the microbiome and body determine something is nonself, it kick starts an immune response. Localized inflammation begins as the heat in the area increases to support the immune cells. The offender is then disarmed and the body can go back to life as usual.

Dr. Junger has a wonderful way of describing this process. There is communication between the gut microbiota and the immune cells, and everything that exists in the body, or comes through the body, is coded. The microbes in the gut actually train our immune system to recognize what is an invader to the body and what isn't. This is ingenious!

Again nature works in a beautiful and efficient fashion. The microbes decide what is friend or foe because they need to create the optimal environment for their survival, and in turn, ours. In Dr. Junger's analogy the immune cells are programmed by the microbiome and act as gatekeepers. When a particle, virus, or whatever else comes up against them, they have a scanner that reads their barcode. The microbes have communicated to the immune cells what the barcodes are, and whether the barcode indicates a substance is friend or foe. If friend, the microbe, particle, or protein is allowed to pass. If foe, the inflammatory, immune response kicks into gear. The interesting thing is that these immune cells are talking to one another across the entire body. Either they get info and travel through the gut to the systemic circulation to lodge in outposts in our arms, legs, and skin, for example, or the cells in those places are getting the intel from the gut cells some other way. In any case, this is how a pathogen that is identified in the gut as foe is recognized the next time it turns up anywhere else in the body, and hopefully is destroyed.

Sometimes autoimmune conditions arise as a result of this natural survival process. The barcode on a pathogen may be so similar to the barcode on a protein in our food, or to one of our own commensal or human cells, that the immune cell's scanner misidentifies friend as foe. In Ayurveda this mistaken identity is viewed as a confusion of the natural intelligence of the body. Just as we humans can feel confused or overwhelmed sometimes, so can the body. This begins the cascade of immune responses that result in the type of systemic or chronic localized inflammation present in autoimmune conditions.

When someone is overeating, overwhelming the GI tract, or eating and thinking and emoting in a way that disturbs metabolic function and microbial balance, digestion doesn't happen optimally. Foods can take too long to digest or not get broken apart and absorbed properly. They just sit around and ferment, feeding bad microbes and creating gasses. Enzymatic activity in the small intestine can diminish, liver and gallbladder function may become sluggish, or the stomach may have too much or not enough acid. Along the way, the valves that the chyme—that mix of partially digested foodstuffs and gastric juices—passes through may lose their timing, so chyme may not be emptied in a timely fashion from the stomach, or valves may not get completely closed. When the food isn't moving through the GI tract fast enough, people will oftentimes complain of feeling like they have a lump in their epigastric region or that they are burping up a meal they ate hours ago. In the small intestine, there can be inflammation that produces too much mucus. Or the intestinal villi, the little finger-like projections covered in even smaller finger-like projections that line the tract, can get flattened, resulting in nutrient malabsorption.

Any or all of these scenarios set the stage for what we deem to be food sensitivities and the signs and symptoms associated with inadequate digestion and assimilation of foods and fluids. In leaky gut syndrome, things that shouldn't get through the gut wall do, and may find their way into the systemic circulation. From an Eastern medicine perspective, when this happens food becomes ama and leads to chronic inflammation. It is sticky (though it can dry out and crust onto tissues), dense, and turbid. It confuses the body and inhibits the flow of communication among cells and other tissues, disturbing nutrient absorption and creation. It also weighs down and further inhibits the digestive process and metabolic processes throughout the body as a whole, depending upon where it spreads. The overall consequences can manifest as pain, malabsorption, skin rashes, fatigue, fogginess, heaviness, lack of motivation, inability to concentrate, depression, and muddled thinking.

This concept is aligned with what happens in the gut and surrounding tissues from a Western science standpoint. Microbes (even friendly ones), food particles, or other metabolites, however tiny, can get through the barriers created by the mucus, epithelial cells, GALT, and commensal bacteria that assist with tight epithelial junctions and the integrity of the mucosal barrier. Here they either trigger localized inflammation and are dealt with; escape beyond the barrier of the GALT deep into the body, lymphatics, or blood; or erroneously encode the immune system with false information that makes the body do strange things, such as lose its intelligent functioning, get confused and attack seemingly harmless substances, or attack itself. Even things that are rightly in the gut can trigger this cascade of events if the integrity of the intestinal barrier is compromised.

What we think and feel affects our ability to keep our body's inherent intelligence on track. For some people these types of disorders can take a lifetime to manifest; in others it happens in the first few years of life. Many people are at different stages of the process, regardless of age or privilege.

Taste's Role in Digestion

Beyond how we eat and what we are feeling affecting our digestion, taste also has a role to play in optimal digestive functioning.

Ayurveda recognizes six primary tastes, and Chinese medicine, five, but taste's role in digestion has been largely ignored in Western medicine. Recently this has begun to change. For example, we now "know" there are taste receptors on the heart for bitter, whereas Chinese medicine has used bitter medicinals for hundreds, if not thousands, of years to balance the heart system.[6]

We recognize that when food has an appealing smell, our digestive juices start flowing, especially if appetite is high. Even the slightest of smells affects our digestion, for better or worse. We also know that even thinking of certain foods, such as a lemon, may cause the mouth to water. Likewise, if we see something unappealing or imagine eating something disgusting, we get the icks and may even feel a bit nauseous. This is the power of the mind influencing digestion.

Once the food is in our mouths, though, the process of digestion immediately begins to affect the whole rest of the body. The taste of the food triggers specific physiological processes. These processes happen in a beneficial yet subtle way in response to substances that nourish and heal us, but we see the adverse effects very clearly with food allergies. If someone with a food allergy ingests that food, or even smells or touches it, the body can start to react.

There are tastes that are considered catabolic, molecule-degrading, or detoxifying; and those that are anabolic, synthesizing, or tissue-building, and necessary for growth. Both are necessary to maintain the health of the body. Some tastes elevate our mental clarity, and some make us feel secure. Some make us feel lighter, some warmer, some cooler. Some have an astringent, squeezing, or holding action for the tissues; some create more movement.

These effects can be quite noticeable, or so subtle you may not even feel them. Results may be noticeable immediately, days later, or after consistent consumption has produced cumulative effects. As mentioned in chapter 1, tastes in the nasal cavity have specific regulating effects on the local immunity. Since they are living beings it makes perfect sense that microbes have some sort of an affinity for taste as well. Carbohydrates have a sweet taste and may nourish some colonies, and the combined sweet and pungent tastes of meats nourish others. The bitter taste of leafy greens may nourish other forms of life, yet in great quantity may be considered hard on some people's digestion due to their rough or cooling qualities. We don't know exact correlations between specific strains of microbes and the five or six tastes and the resultant effects on the mind and body, but we do know that certain communities thrive when specific types of macromolecules and their resultant tastes predominate. For example, some microbial entities thrive when there are large amounts of meat and fat in the diet, and others thrive when a varied abundance of fruits and vegetables is consumed. Those with a predominance of meat and fat in their diets are found to have gut microbiomes predominant in communities linked to higher rates of inflammation and obesity, and those with diets high in vegetable matter, including grains, with communities associated with the opposite.

Beyond a few examples, which are like drops of water in a sea of information, we haven't scientifically confirmed the correlations between taste, specific foods, and microbial colonies. However, from an

Eastern medicine perspective we have what tastes do in the body down to a science. The terms *microbes, beneficial bacteria,* and *microbiome* may not be part of the Eastern medicine vocabulary, but the concept of the microbiome, largely based on knowing what it does, is refined. Innumerable texts, ancient and modern, describe what to eat for each mind-body type or condition, and what not to eat. There is also specific information detailing how and when to eat, based on thousands of years of insight. These directives can be found in Egyptian hieroglyphs, the foundational writings of Hippocrates, and in the source texts of all Eastern medicines.

What Goes In—and How

Food can be medicine and can create medicinal effects in the body and mind. We are now understanding another facet to these actions from a Western science perspective, and that is through the action of the microbiome and its metabolites. What we are seeing is that when you eat something, your mental state, the smell of the food, your thoughts and feelings about the food, and whatever else is going on in you at that moment all affect your digestion. If you feel bad about what you're eating, or if you shame yourself for it afterward, it negatively impacts how that meal gets metabolized.

Since the microbiome helps digest food and provides nutrients, it is also part of the digestive process and GI tract. We don't know everything about how our thoughts and feelings affect the microbiome, but we know that they affect how we digest our food. It stands to reason that how we feel impacts the microbiome, since we know that how we feel affects our physiology. There is plenty of research to show how negatively an excessive stress response impacts our body, and since the microbiome is part of our body, it would only make sense that it too would be adversely affected by how we experience or react to stressors. Travel across time zones, trauma, and illness all create dysbiosis in the microbiome. The effects of specific mental ruminations on the microbiome have not been studied, but we know when we feel good and when we don't. We know if we feel lousy after we eat certain things or when we think certain things. If feeling a certain way secretes molecules that the body's cells respond to, then why wouldn't those same messages from the brain affect the microbiome? Digestion begins in the mind, and also physiologically in the brain. Smell affects the brain, and this sends signals to the rest of the body. Tastes also create systemic effects.

The food we chew mixes with saliva, which contains enzymes, then enters the stomach, where it gets sloshed around and further prepared for digestion. In Eastern medicine we say not to put food on top of food. This is because it overwhelms the body's intelligence and capacity to digest well. If food is ingested and an hour later more is eaten, most likely the earlier food is still in there "rotting and ripening." When this happens the new food starts to rot as well, but not ripen. What's better is for the digestive process to happen in stages, so that the breakdown and subsequent fermentation are clean and uninhibited.

When the process is hampered by overwhelming the body, it makes it difficult for the whole lot to be digested properly. This can lead to a feeling like a rock in the stomach, or an ache, nausea, indigestion, heartburn, or burping. The stomach intelligently decides the order of processing what is consumed. Fluids go through the stomach first, followed by the solid food. A presentation I attended at Seattle Institute of East Asian Medicine indicated that meat or protein should be eaten first. The rationale behind this was that the highest concentration of acid would go to digesting that first, since it takes a long time to digest, whereas later in the meal the acid would be less concentrated and less efficient. I don't know if this is true, as I've also heard the opposite: easier to digest foods in first, because they can be more quickly liquefied for the small intestine. I lean toward the first opinion, protein first, and encourage you to try it for yourself. In Italy, it is common to have salad at the end of a meal, not the beginning. This catches my attention since I have had many clients who've come back from there, where they have often eaten day in and day out. Yet they remark on how well their digestion worked despite the lengthy meals. Better than at home. One reason for this is that they have different wheat in Italy, but the other, I suspect, is the order in which they eat.

Another consideration in deciding what to put into the body—and how—is the concept of food combining. We hear about this in Western nutrition, and it's also a premise in Eastern traditions. There are foods that don't digest well together, yet in our culture we combine them all the time: eggs and cheese, yogurt and fruit, bread and meat, melon and anything, even other types of fruit. The primary emphasis in Western thought is that it is best not to pair proteins and carbs, and that's pretty much as far as most people's exposure to this concept goes. Maybe that doesn't even sound familiar to you. Even though this is what may be recommended, what happens with a sandwich or a burger? Chronic poor food combinations are a recipe for generating ama, or toxins. The quick, comfort, go-to items in a typical Western diet, which are primary choices in our increasingly demanding lives, are less than ideal when it comes to encouraging optimal digestion. When something digests well, we should not be experiencing a food coma; we should actually feel light and energized after we eat. We should feel satiated, satisfied, comfortable, grounded, and full of energy. How often can you say that happens to you?

More frequently the norm is to feel an awareness of digestion, tired, heavy, mentally dull, sluggish, and craving caffeine or sweets. There may be abdominal discomfort, acidity, feeling mucusy, full, bloated, or like the food is stuck in the epigastric area. These are all indications that something isn't right. Correct food combining will help remedy this situation, as will eating at regular mealtimes. Human mammals are part of the animal kingdom, and if you've ever had a dog or cat, you know how much they rely on their routines, and yours. They know when it's time to eat and they let you know it very clearly. The human body is the same way. It has a sense of timing, and it needs to be nurtured as much as your beloved pet.

Regular mealtimes shouldn't occur before a minimum of three to four hours following the prior meal. I think even this is pushing it. Unless you're hypoglycemic or have some other medical condition that requires more frequent eating, I recommend four to six hours between meals. This allows enough time for the small intestine to sweep away any leftover debris. Ever noticed your tummy grumble a few hours after eating? That is the sound of the small intestine cleaning itself. It literally clears out *everything* from the previous meal, every particle.

Each time we eat there is a subtle inflammatory process that occurs. This allows for greater blood flow to the intestines for extraction and absorption of nutrients. The increased attention to the gut lining also allows for immune cells in the GALT to be on alert for what's incoming. If you're eating every two hours or snacking, drinking shakes, or sipping coffees with cream and sugar, you are potentially reinflaming the GI tract. This inflammation serves a purpose when meals are at a good interval, four to six hours apart. In Ayurveda we say the stomach should be one-third food, one-third fluid, and one-third air, with the fluid coming mostly from the food, along with some sips of hot water. That's the perfect ratio for optimal combustion. Digestive fire (*agni*) needs air and operates in a medium of fluid (watery element*), so as to not create excess inflammation or burn the mucosal lining.

Once the food moves from the stomach to the small intestine, bile and enzymes start their job in the process of digestion. Bile salts from the liver and gallbladder that are released into the small intestine help us metabolize fats and absorb fat-soluble vitamins. Bile also carries with it wastes and toxins that the liver has cleaned from the blood to be eliminated from the body through the digestive tube.

Enzymes secreted by the pancreas and small intestine further break down the macromolecules of fats, proteins, and carbs. However, if you drink a lot of fluids before you eat, especially iced or cold water, it dilutes or inhibits the enzymatic activity in the small intestine.

*For more information on the elements of Eastern medicine, see "Understanding the Five Elements" on page 64.

Keep It Warm

Regardless of time of year, in Eastern medicine it is contraindicated to consume iced drinks. The body requires warmth for good communication in the tissues, for movement, and for transformation or chemical reactions. Cold is contracting, inhibiting, and congealing, which is not desirable for an environment that is full of fluids constantly needing to move. It's not good for digestion, proper pace of movement, or enzymatic concentration. Consider this: When you wash grease off your dinner dishes, do you use cold or hot water? Hot water, of course, because the heat encourages the grease to melt off instead of stick. This is a good metaphor to use for your insides, particularly concerning the parts responsible for fat metabolism.

This influence cold has over enzymes may well be a primary reason why Eastern medicine recommends eating cooked foods. We have evolved over millennia to do so. When food is cooked, it saves the body energy because it's partially predigested. When proteins are cooked, for example, they are already being broken down by the heat, which makes it easier for the body to do its work. This is particularly important for air/wind/*vata* types, those with *vishama agni*, or irregular metabolism, and those with spleen qi deficiency, or digestive weakness. (See more about metabolic typing in chapter 3.)

Once food enters the small intestine there is a lot of activity. The aforementioned barcode cataloguing, raw material breakdown, nutrient absorption, and systemic detoxification ensues. It is a very busy, fast-paced environment. Transit time of food in the small intestine is much faster than in the large intestine, potentially only five or six hours. How does it do so much in so little time? One answer might be surface area. The folds of the small intestine increase its surface area, as do its finger-like villi, allowing for greater absorption. Healthy villi are adequately supplied with blood, but when villi become swollen or flattened due to certain inflammatory diseases, it interferes with the absorption of nutrients and can even be life-threatening.

During this process the small intestine has a cycle of movement patterns that help slosh the food around, mixing it with fluid, bile, and enzymes. There are four stages to this activity that goes through 90 to 120-minute cycles. One part is a period of no contraction. The next, unsynchronized contractions. Then strong contractions move the food down the tract, followed by the housekeeper phase that cleans out small debris and microbes that don't belong. If any phase is disrupted, if contractions are irregular when they should be regular, or if the muscle tissue is weak, as is the case with issues like scleroderma, the contractions cannot occur as they should, and food and microbes can build up and create imbalance.[7]

Most studies on the microbiome have focused on the flora in the large intestine, specifically, the bacteria. As time goes on, more studies are being carried out on the microbes in the small intestine, and what they are finding is very interesting.

One such study, published in April 2018, showed that small intestine microbes play a significant role in the digestion and absorption of fats.[8] For the study, sterile mice were given a high-fat diet. You may be wondering what sterile rodents have to do with the small intestine microbiome. Quite a bit, actually. These mice weren't sexually sterile but had sterile guts, meaning no gut microbiomes. When they were fed high-fat diets, they didn't metabolize the lipids well and passed them in their stool. Nonsterile mice—ones that had gut microbiomes—developed an abundance of a particular species of microbe that digests fats, and it made them fat. When the sterile mice were administered the fat-metabolizing microbes, they gained the ability to deal with fats. Given there's only so much surface to colonize, an increase in these microbes from the Clostridiaceae and Peptostreptococcaceae families led to a decrease in other microbial communities, including those from the Bifidobacteriaceae and Bacteroidaceae families. These are the ones associated with being lean.[9]

This was just one study, funded by the National Institutes of Health, and it raised many questions and avenues for further exploration: Just how much do our bile and enzymes contribute to fat metabolism, and what are their roles in the presence of these microbes? Do we need less bile and enzymes to digest fats if we have an abundance of these communities in the upper real estate of the gut? Is it possible that liver/gallbladder congestion or sludge in the gallbladder is partially a result of a dysbiosis among fat metabolizing microbial species? The lead author of the study also proposed the possibility of developing postbiotics.[10] These would be supplements containing bacterially derived compounds or metabolites, as opposed to prebiotics (nourishment for the microbes), or probiotics (the microbes themselves). These findings, and the potential of postbiotics, present the possibility of modifying the small bowel ecosystem in an effort to combat obesity, and amending the functioning of the large bowel in chronic inflammatory conditions. It could even affect the performance of extra–alimentary canal digestive organs, such as the pancreas.[11]

The large intestine houses the greatest concentration of microbes in the GI tract, and to date most research done on the microbiome has been on the bacterial strains of the large intestine. In fact, when someone uses the terminology, *gut microbiome,* what they are generally referring to is the one in the large intestine. The synergy of its cells and the microbes inhabiting it allow for us to extract, create, and absorb such important nutrients as fatty acids and vitamins. The dreaded E. coli bacteria, when in balanced quantity in the right place, is actually a helpful part of the gut microbiome, responsible for the production of vitamin K. Lactic acid microbes, such as bifidobacteria, can synthesize necessary vitamins we cannot make ourselves. These include the vitamins B12, riboflavin, thiamine, and folate. It makes me wonder why so many people need supplementation of these. Do they lack the food needed by the bifidobacteria, or lack the bifidobacteria themselves? Is some step in the process of breaking down the food, or communication between cells and microbes causing the problem? Is the culprit some kind of circulation or absorption issue?

The appendix is immune tissue that also acts as a warehouse for good bacteria. In addition to detecting and ridding the body of potentially harmful microbes, researchers have found that its stored beneficial microbes can repopulate the gut in the aftermath of a bout of diarrhea. This keeps communities we don't want from setting up shop in the available space on the gut wall.[12] The large intestine microbiome is a vast subject, because it is where the vast majority of our microbes live.

SCFAs: The Beauty of Butyrate

When talking about the large intestine microbiome it's important to mention that in addition to the production of vitamins, these microbes feed on fiber to produce short chain fatty acids (SCFAs). Short chain fatty acids can reduce the effects of stress on our gut and behavior.

Butyrate, a type of SCFA, is produced by the fermentation of resistant starch (that is, it resists digestion), an important food source for "friendly" bacteria in the colon. Dietary fiber passes undigested through the stomach and small intestine and ferments in the large intestine, feeding that microbiome. Here SCFAs are created from the resistant starches by the resident microbes and used as an energy source for the human cells that line the lower intestine. Although it's not yet clear how it works, a 2018 study showed the introduction of these SCFAs resulted in decreased levels of stress and anxiety-like behavior.

Butyrate has numerous other benefits, including the following: it decreases or even prevents colonic inflammation and leads to destruction of colon cancer cells, enhances intestinal membrane health, helps to repair the epithelial cells of the innermost lining in the gut, and increases mucosal integrity. In animal studies, it increased absorption of minerals.[13] It protects the intestinal barrier by increasing production of mucin,[14] a gel-like substance that coats the inside of the gut; and can actually help repair leaky gut, which is often a result of stress. It affects the immune response by assisting neutrophil migration to inflammatory sites, thus increasing apopto-sis (self-destruction of damaged cells) and decreasing cell growth.[15] Antimicrobial peptides are also increased due to butyrate.[16]

Butyrate has been found to work best in low concentrations and may actually work against the integrity of the gut wall in too high a dosage, which is why I wouldn't run out and buy it as a supple-ment. A well-balanced, high-fiber diet is the best course of action.[17] In addition to its protective mechanisms in the large intestine, butyr-ate increases insulin sensitivity and glucose tolerance.[18] It can cross the blood-brain barrier, activating the hypothalamus and vagus nerve, affecting appetite and eating behavior. Via the gut-brain axis it also affects host metabolism by enhancing the proportion of nerves regu-lating gut motility.[19]

What Comes Out—and When

The time it takes for food to move through the digestive tract varies depending on a number of issues: what was eaten, how much, psychologi-cal factors, and even gender. Different foods travel at different rates, and not necessarily in the order eaten. Estimates for how long food remains in a healthy stomach range anywhere from forty-five minutes to six hours. In response to a question posed on the Mayo Clinic's website, one doc-tor commented that transit time from the stomach through the intes-tines averages more than fifty hours. It takes about six to eight hours to get through the small intestine, so the bulk of that time is spent in the large intestine. In a study cited from the 1980s, the transit time through the large intestine averaged thirty-three hours for men and forty-seven hours for women.[20] That's a lot of time for food to be in your body! Giulia Enders, M.D., author of *Gut: The Inside Story of Our Body's Most Underrated Organ,* disagrees with those time estimates. She believes the time it takes for food to be processed in the large intestine is about six-teen hours.[21] Whatever the case, food is in us for quite a while. If it moves too quickly, we may not be absorbing enough nutrients and water. Too slow, and the extra fermentation time may create excessive gas, bloating, and constipation. Functional medicine doctors and holistic practitioners agree that the transit time should be less than quoted above, and most advocate that a healthy length of time for the entire process from mouth to toilet should be twelve to twenty-four hours.

There is a lot of conflicting information regarding transit times and what constitutes healthy intestinal function, and it's difficult to know what to believe. I propose getting to know your own body's transit time. Know that it may change based on what you've eaten. Eat some beets and make a note of what time it is. When you see reddish stool in the toilet, assuming of course there is no bleeding, then you know how long it took for it to get through. This is a general idea of transit time, at least for beets. Things like red meat take longer, perhaps days, whereas liquids move more quickly. If the beet test doesn't work for you, you could try taking activated charcoal, which causes black stool. The charcoal is also a good detoxifier, but be sure to heed any health warnings on the label.

My proposal is that we listen, feel, and experiment. Listen to what our instincts and intuition tell us about the food that is most beneficial for us, how we feel when we eat, and when we eat certain things. It's another way to know ourselves better. It requires that we stop fixating on taking in information and instead tap into what feels right in our bodies. This is a tricky switch to flip. We are accustomed to ignoring the body, mind-over-matter, so to speak. But the body is speaking to us all the time. We get feelings, inclinations, hunches, dreams, a sense of something, a sixth sense, premonitions, and instinctive alerts. These often get stuffed down, rationalized, or ignored, since they often defy logic and our culture values thought and logic more than intuition. Yet how much better do you feel in your skin when you create a balance between reason and feeling? It can take practice to be a good listener or it can happen in an instant, and it is imperative to our well-being, our homeostasis, and prevention of disease. In the case of the microbiome, listening or not can affect not only our physical health, but our mental and emotional life.

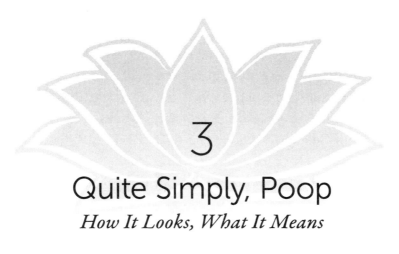

3

Quite Simply, Poop
How It Looks, What It Means

Everyone poops.

TARO GOMI,
CHILDREN'S BOOK AUTHOR

We can't talk about the microbiome without talking about poop. The quality, quantity, and timing of bowel movements is an important diagnostic tool in both modern and traditional medicines. It reflects the quality of the gut wall environment, metabolic type of the individual, health of accessory digestive organ functioning, and potentially the adequate diversity and health of the microbiome.

Poop as Medicine

Did you know poop is medicinal? The first recorded instance of using stool for therapeutic purposes was in fourth-century China, where Chinese medical doctor Ge Hong had patients with dysentery-like disorders drink a concoction called "yellow soup." The main ingredient? You guessed it: poop. Stool was prepared in different ways in order to treat varying patterns of bowel disharmony. Later, another Chinese doctor, Li Shi Zhen, made his own version of the recipe and called it "golden syrup." It was a combination of fresh, fermented, and dried stool. He expanded its thera-peutic applicability by using it to treat a variety of ailments ranging from diarrhea to constipation as well as fever, pain, and—get this—vomiting.[1] Eastern medicine had a major leg up on fecal microbiota transplantation, or FMT, with Ge Hong's creation and Li Shi Zhen's modifications. The procedure was used for some time in China, but eventually fell out of vogue, arguably due to distaste. Eastern medicine practitioners are still taught about these remedies because they weren't just weird, they were effective. Today, Western medicine is avidly researching the use of poop as a therapeutic agent.

Bodily waste remedies are not restricted to human byproducts. For example, flying squirrel turds are highly valued in Chinese medicine for their usefulness in treating blood stasis, postpartum abdominal pain, retained lochia (discharge following vaginal birth), and some forms of childhood nutritional impairment. In North Africa, Bedouins have long used fresh, warm camel poop to cure diarrheal diseases.

In Chinese medicine, the urine of prepubescent boys is highly prized for invigorating the blood and helping restore strength to depleted post-partum women. It may be that the hormones in the urine account for its medicinal effects, or maybe it's the microbial makeup, or some combina-tion of both. Whatever the mechanism of action underlying urine as a medicinal substance, it is an annual spring tradition in the Chinese city of Dongyang to consume eggs cooked in young boys' urine. Collection buckets are lined up in the halls of Chinese elementary schools to sup-ply the cooking medium. "Virgin boy eggs" are believed to increase energy, decrease excess body heat, and regulate circulation.

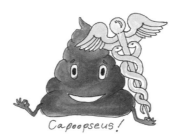

Medicinal poop emoji

Capoopseus!

In Ayurveda, cow urine is considered a remedy for cough, some skin and eye diseases, and diarrhea, and is also said to strengthen the brain. *Panchagavya,* a mixture of cow dung, urine, milk, yogurt, and ghee, is a potent detoxifier and immune booster. Cow dung is also burned to clear the air of pathogens, as it is prized for its antimicrobial properties. Cow dung and butter can be used as a potion to treat ulcers, or can be combined with cow urine for treating wheezing and coughing. The pressed juice from the combination can be used to treat many abdominal complaints.[2] But what is it in cow dung that has all these miraculous benefits? It is rich in nutritive substances, and research on it is being carried out as a potential treatment for antibiotic-resistant strains of bacteria in humans. But don't run out to collect dung from the nearest farm anytime soon; according to one study, the benefits are most present in cows indigenous to, and located in, India.[3]

In veterinary medicine, the stool of various animals has been used for halting diarrhea for decades. Modern use of stool as medicine officially reemerged in the 1950s. This happened when a doctor documented successfully using retention enemas of fecal transplant material for treatment of antibiotic-associated diarrhea.

In humans, fecal microbiota transplantation (FMT) is a procedure by which feces are prepared in a lab and administered either orally or rectally, most often by colonoscopy in severe cases of illness. It wasn't until 1978 that fecal transplants became widely accepted in treating *Clostridium difficile* (C. diff.) infections, with a cure rate of 95 percent.[4] C. diff is a bacterial infection that causes potentially life-threatening diarrhea. FMT is considered an accepted treatment for C. diff infection, but regulation has stiffened. The words *transplant* and *donor* are appropriate terminology for the practice since it's widely accepted as a form of organ transplant—the microbiome organ—so physicians are required to go through an approval process; currently it is approved only for treatment of C. diff. Studies are currently underway for potential treatment of disorders ranging from gastrointestinal issues to autism spectrum disorder and Alzheimer's disease.

Because of its efficacy and uncertainty about long-term side effects, human poop is now classified as a pharmaceutical agent. This bans use without a prescription, and there is slim chance of obtaining one. The strict regulations on FMT don't stop some people, though. Those with a range of disorders are taking it upon themselves to find perceivably healthy donors in a desperate attempt to self-heal their guts, metabolic syndromes, mental/emotional disorders, or obesity issues. Others have started legitimate labs that collect samples for regulated FMT. The non-profit OpenBiome requires rigorous screening of blood and stool over a number of weeks, and 75 percent of samples are rejected. Most rejections are due to international travel, recent antibiotic usage, or certain microbes, but the lucky few who are accepted get paid $40 a sample.[5]

Human poop is an amazing diagnostic tool for Eastern and Western medicine practitioners alike, but what exactly is it? Under a microscope our waste is found to be made up of microbes (alive and dead), sloughed epithelial cells, mucus, and digested and undigested food.[6] Some sources say it contains up to one-third dead bacteria. Stool contains quite a bit of water, as well as fats, salts, a tiny bit of protein, and whatever was released into the intestines from the liver. Contrary to popular vernacular, the scent doesn't come from roses; it's largely a byproduct of sulfur-containing foods, microbes producing sulfur-containing compounds, and hydrogen sulfide. Most of the gassy smell is produced by anaerobic microbes breaking down proteins.[7]

A Raleigh, North Carolina, not-for-profit called the Rome Foundation was designed to create international collaboration and consensus of scientific data for diagnosis and treatment of functional GI disorders, and also disseminates information to the general public on how to manage functional GI disorders.[8] They recommend the Bristol Stool Form Scale, which is utilized internationally by gastroenterologists in stool assessment and is the accepted standard in poop analysis. It classifies the health of stool in a range of seven categories, from hard pellets to watery diarrhea.

BRISTOL STOOL CHART

Type 1 — Separate hard lumps — SEVERE CONSTIPATION

Type 2 — Lumpy and Sausage like — MILD CONSTIPATION

Type 3 — Sausage Shaped with cracks in the Surface — NORMAL

Type 4 — Like a Smooth Soft Sausage or Snake ~ Floaters! — NORMAL

Type 5 — Soft blobs with clear-cut edges — LACKING FIBRE

Type 6 — Mushy Consistency with ragged edges — LOOSE STOOL

Type 7 — Liquid Consistency with no Solid Pieces — DIARRHEA

The Bristol Stool Chart, or Bristol Stool Form Scale, is the accepted standard in stool analysis.

Poop Diagnosis in Eastern Medicine

Eastern medicine recognizes that the environment in the intestines needs to be "just so" in order for digestion to function optimally and produce healthy bowel movements. The appearance of the feces reflects that environment, and it provides diagnostic information about other organs and the individual as a whole. The intestines should not be too dry, too hot, or too wet. The nervous system should be regulated so that there aren't timing issues associated with peristalsis. Optimal stool is formed; contains no undigested food particles, mucus, or blood; is the shape of the colon, tapered at the ends; is easy to pass; comes out completely on a regular schedule; is medium brown, not pale, not dark; and doesn't stick to the toilet bowl. Some even say it should float a bit and the smell should be minimal. This is fairly congruent with the Western analysis, although the Bristol model leaves room for variation as to what is ideal. In Eastern assessment we are much more specific in that only one type of stool on the chart is considered ideal (type 4). Using information about the stool we are able to identify subclinical patterns that, if treated properly, may never manifest clinically. Changes in diet, travel, stress, lack of sleep, and change in water consumption can all affect the stool.

Poop is very important in Eastern medicine. It tells us a lot about what's happening internally, and how to treat it. The large intestine is important for absorbing water, forming stools, and eliminating waste and toxins. In Ayurveda the channels that eliminate metabolic waste and toxins are called *mala srotas.* In Chinese medicine the large intestine, *da chang,* receives the products of the small intestine and eliminates waste in tandem with the lungs. Regularity is key, preferably once a day upon waking. It shouldn't be an urgent bowel movement, nor difficult to pass. Twice a day is also acceptable, once upon waking and additionally after a meal.

People often report a formed bowel movement in the morning, then later on they pass one that's loose, but this second loose stool is not ideal. It may have at its root a deficiency, cold or heat, and is usually associated with caffeine consumption. Many people rely on caffeine for elimination. Caffeine, and in particular, coffee, is an addiction when one relies upon it for stimulation to evacuate. People who are in this boat are usually burning the candle at both ends—tired, overworked, or too busy to not be drinking caffeine. I encourage people to at least temporarily remove caffeine, namely coffee, from their diets to get a handle on their baseline for energy and bowel health. It can be a trying process, but being honest with oneself about what is happening and rebalancing is better for long-term health. It is amazing what people notice when they let go of the need for caffeine, especially coffee.

The Bristol chart explains stool in terms of constipation, diarrhea, and the variable normalcy between those extremes. Constipation can range from not going at all for days to having daily or multiple-a-day bowel movements that are incomplete. If you feel like you're done and you're still wiping stool onto the toilet paper repeatedly, that is also a form of constipation. This scenario may fall under a lack of vitality, where there is a sluggishness on the way out of the colon, or dampness in the colon. A deficiency of vitality or a qi deficiency can also manifest as having an urge to defecate, but the person can't go and feels bloated. Dampness and toxins are synonymous. Dampness/ama is a bogginess in the body that gums up the works and creates a range of issues from brain fog to sensations of heaviness. Stools heavy in dampness tend to stick to the toilet bowl.

Metabolic Typing according to Poop Analysis

Ayurveda classifies stool patterns into metabolic types that are associated with imbalances in the doshas, or mind-body constitutional profiles, which are a reflection of the five elements, or building blocks of matter and how it behaves. When the intestinal lining is too dry, this is called *vishama agni,* meaning the metabolism is irregular. It is caused by abundant vata dosha, or a dry, cold, mobility-dominant constitution, and is associated mostly with the air element. The stool tends to be dark brown, irregular, scanty, dry or hard, bulletlike, and difficult to pass. Passing it may include pain, it has an astringent odor, and it sinks quickly in the toilet. This metabolic type may be prone to constipation, gas, bloating, food intolerance, fatigue after eating, anxiety, fear, dry skin, poor sleep, and joint issues. A vata tongue may be small, pale, or dry with scalloped edges and a quiver. It is recommended to balance the air element of the body by relaxing around mealtimes; eating at regularly scheduled mealtimes; eating warm, cooked foods; leaning toward sweet, sour, and salty tastes; and incorporating more oils and fats into the diet. Recommended spices and teas to help with this include ginger, cardamom, cumin, fennel, coriander, and licorice root.

Understanding the Five Elements

The five elements of Eastern medicine may be, for simplicity of understanding, likened to the periodic table in chemistry. They are the building blocks of matter and have specific traits and tendencies that describe how matter, and nature, behaves. Five element theory describes how everything interacts—for instance, how one substance may increase or decrease, nourish or aggravate, another. Those who laid the foundations of Eastern medicine recognized patterns, signs, symptoms, traits, activities, behaviors, reactions, manifestations, and actions that are the sum of all the substances and processes of the human body. They categorized these into the traits that make up the elements and their activities. These include the existence and actions of the microbes within us, so when we say something is due to excess fire, for example, there may be a specific microbe, set of microbes, or metabolites working in concert with our cells and metabolic processes that create symptoms of heat in the body and mind. Eastern medicine practitioners are trained to recognize those signs and symptoms, diagnose their cause, and determine how to not only alleviate the symptoms but address the cause using various therapies. One of the primary diagnostic tools we utilize is stool diagnosis.

The metabolic type associated with imbalanced pitta dosha, or a hot, transformative-dominant constitution, is called *tikshna agni* and signifies sharp, quick, hot, or hypermetabolism. It is caused by an excess of the fire element. Those with hypermetabolism can have a voracious appetite and get irritated if they are hungry. They may crave sweets; be prone to reflux; suffer from bad breath or body odor; anger easily; have hot flashes, blood sugar issues, and skin rashes; and experience nausea and liver and gallbladder* issues. Their tongues may be smooth, wet,

---

*The organs in Eastern medicine have a very different meaning than in Western medicine. Although their definitions do for the greater part incorporate the structure and function we are accustomed to hearing about, they encompass much more. Each organ is not just a part of the body, but an entire system that contributes to and intimately interacts with everything else within us. The organs have physical and psychic roles in the body-mind whole.

and reddish. Their bowel movements may be urgent, hot, loose, soft, liquidy, and fall apart easily. To balance out the excess fire they should favor fresh foods, including fruits and veggies. Ghee and coconut oils are recommended to some extent, as well as the sweet and bitter tastes. Cilantro is good, as is mint tea.

Dull or hypometabolism is called *munda agni* and is associated with kapha dosha, or the moist, stability-dominant constitutional type. Dull or hypometabolism is a digestive process that gets bogged down by the heaviness, density, coolness, and wetness of the earth and water elements. Those with this type of metabolism need to counteract it with more fire element, and also the lightness and movement of air. They may have longer transit times and their digestive process overall is long, heavy, and slow. They can gain weight easily, feel tired a lot, and feel a sense of heaviness after eating. They may experience mild water retention, clammy skin, or circulatory issues, and be prone to lymphatic congestion, excessive mucus production, and phlegm congestion. Their bowel movements tend to be sticky and sluggish, large, copious, heavy, oily, and on the pale side, but usually well formed and regular. Stools can smell sickly sweet. The tongue may be puffy, dense, slightly scalloped, greasy or slimy, and have a thick coating. Adding more spices, salty, pungent, and warming foods may help to balance the dull, heavy qualities associated with hypometabolism. Fermented foods can be good, as well as ginger and pepper.

Balanced digestion, or *sama agni* is achievable for any of the constitutional types in a state of good health. Hunger arises naturally, not in excess, but also not absent. There is a pleasant anticipation of eating and the foods that are eaten satisfy the hunger. There is a feeling of lightness and clarity after meals, and the mind tends to be clear, calm, content, and happy. Those with balanced digestion can digest most foods, within reason. They tolerate seasonal change well, have good immunity, and zero discomfort after eating. Their bowel movements happen one to two times daily, a few minutes after waking and again later after a meal. The stool is well formed, the consistency of a ripe banana. It is brown, maintains its shape, is only slightly oily, has only a mild odor, and doesn't immediately sink or stick to the toilet. There is no stickiness on the toilet paper either.

We can explain the principles of metabolic typing from the Ayurvedic tradition alongside those of Chinese medicine. Stomach heat and heat in general is a causative factor in many bowel irregularities, particularly present in patterns of constipation, and often combines with dryness. Constipation that is blatant or severe, often accompanied by infrequent bowel movements, pain, and gas, is usually due to dryness and/or heat in the system. We can also say this is a *vata* type of stool, since vata is dry and causes dryness. Heat consumes fluids and can also create dryness, so although the stools may be dry, they can have a heat or a *pitta* imbalance at their root. Sometimes heated stools will be hard as well as dry, and the person may experience thirstiness, bad breath, and fullness in the abdomen. Heat in the large intestine can also make the stool dark and malodorous.

Heat and dampness may mix in the system and may manifest as loose bowel movements and create a sense of rectal heaviness and urge to evacuate (tenesmus), or there may be yellow mucus in the stool. Any mucus in the stool is attributed to an imbalance of *kapha,* or a dull metabolism. Dampness and heat mixing can also cause increased frequency of bowel movements, burning sensations, and thirstiness. If there is liver qi stagnation, that is, holding due to fear or stress, there will be constipation with pellet-like stools. Liver-spleen disharmony creates stress reactivity or tension that taxes the ability of the body to transform food and fluids. In this case, bowel movements can alternate between being loose and dry, or may be irregular.

We generally associate loose bowel movements with damaged *pitta* in Ayurveda. This would be considered a fast metabolism or things moving through the digestive tract too quickly due to heat or inflammation. In Chinese medicine we'd say the spleen qi is damaged, and that a deficiency of qi can lead to faulty transformation. When this is the case, the stool can have a fishy odor and there may be pain present. Cold mixed with dampness can cause loose bowels or watery diarrhea, may be pale yellow, foul smelling, and there may be fullness of the abdomen and pain. Cold and pain usually go together in Eastern medicine. Blood deficiency, due to either anemia or preclinical blood deficiency, can cause hard or dry stools. If the vitality is so depleted that there is debilitating yang deficiency, then the situation is very serious and the person has totally undigested food moving through and out of the body. Yang is the source physiological heat and energy that the body needs to survive, and is the foundational support for the function of the spleen qi.

Enterotypes

As we've explored above, the inner gut ecology varies from individual to individual. Each person's microbiome is as unique as their human genetic makeup. In spite of our inherent individuality, there are still ways to categorize people that help us to understand their traits or tendencies, predispositions, and potential medical treatment options. One example of this is how, as different as we all are, we all have a specific blood type category we fall into. Some researchers have found this to be the case with the gut microbiome as well. Although the categories are changeable and more overlapping than distinct, having somewhat clear groupings is helpful for scientists for a number of reasons. It can help us better understand the relationship between microbiome types and physiological tendencies. It can help us better understand a person's metabolism, and potentially the likelihood of developing certain diseases, how the person could be treated, and the potential response to treatment. We aren't there yet, but researchers have recognized the likelihood of microbiome types.

In Eastern medicine we call definable trait groupings of body types constitutions. As an extension of constitution, we recognize digestive processing types, as explained in the previous section. In Western medicine there is a concept of gut microbiome types that dictate the potential for an individual's metabolism, physique, and overall health. These microbial types are called *enterotypes*.

When researchers first published Western findings on enterotypes there were several classifications. Upon reading this I got very excited because I thought they must perfectly align with Eastern medicine constitutional classifications. In Ayurveda there are three predominant classifications, and in Chinese medicine there are five. However, after further research I found they are lumped into two groupings. Okay, not ideal for my mind that likes to make simple connections, but still very interesting. Those two gut microbiome types are dominated by either *Bacteroides* or *Prevotella* bacteria. Since the time it was decided there are only two enterotypes, the discussion has reopened to the possibility that there are indeed more. These types are not cut and dry but rather overlap. Although dominance can be in one type, the other types are still present. Researchers are also finding that the dominant gut microbes change depending upon where a person is in the life cycle. This is aligned with Eastern medicine teachings about constitution. Right now, since the scientific community is talking mostly about the *Bacteroides* and *Prevotella* enterotypes, we will focus on those here. I'm hoping they will further diversify the classifications after more studies are completed.

Bacteroides types, as mentioned in the introduction to this book, are those whose diets are high in meats and fats; they tend to have less diverse microbiomes and greater incidence of inflammation and obesity. The typical *Prevotella* diet is richer in fiber, including carbohydrates and sugars, with microbiomes that tend toward greater diversity and are correlated with a leaner physique and less inflammation. Given that information, most people would probably hope to fall into the *Prevotella*-dominant enterotype. There have been a slew of studies changing people's diets and testing their microbiomes to see if enterotype change is possible, and if so, permanent. So far researchers have found that it is indeed possible, temporarily. But even after six months of diet change, once the individual goes back to their regular diet, their enterotype changes back to what it was. This could be because of food choices, but it could also be because our enterotype is more than what we eat. Somehow, microbial communities are passed down through the generations as well. It may be there is much more to this story of how we are seeded and how changeable it is. I suspect investigating this process and having more answers to this may also answer questions about how to create probiotics that are able to take root rather than just pass through the system.

Probiotics

Knowing what good stools are and being able to see when they're less than desirable can be unsettling. It's not uncommon to want to find a solution to unbalanced digestion by jumping on the latest diet trend and fasting, doing a liver flush, or reaching for supplements. We all want to feel better and will often go to great lengths to do so. There is a tendency to believe the latest trends due to the hope that the latest thing is the panacea we've been waiting for all along. One of those new crowd-pleasing solutions is probiotics.

Probiotics are supplements containing microbes believed to be beneficial. There are also *prebiotics,* or supplements that contain food for microbes as opposed to the microbes themselves, and *postbiotics,* or supplements containing the products of microbes that help our bodies stay well. Although they are not living microbes, the potential for these are promising, and in some instances they may be more suited to people with certain medical conditions or to people in underdeveloped countries, as there is less fuss with preservation and shelf life. *Psychobiotics* are more like probiotics in that they contain live microbes, but the contents are specific to those that confer a proven mental wellness benefit. *Synbiotics* are supplements that contain a combination of pre and probiotics.

Probiotics are taken most often during a course of antibiotics, for vaginal health, to promote healthy bowel movements, and to make dairy products more easily digestible by those with lactose intolerance. Probiotic supplements are big business, one that will expand over the coming years as more and more of the population become aware of their microbiomes. One probiotic market trend report projects an increased demand over the next several years, and cites that a *Lactobacillus* strain (although they didn't state which one) alone was valued at 1.2 billion dollars in 2017.[9]

What do probiotics do? That's still up for debate and requires more research. Ideally, they help to balance the immune system and other factors in the body on their journey through you. They may be alive or dead when you ingest them and by the time they exit. Think of it like this: the more you take, the more you'll poop out. It is a fairly common misconception that the microbes in probiotics stick around and create a new home for themselves in our bodies. As far as we know, with the strains and supplements we currently have at our disposal, this is not true. Although taking probiotics may be a good temporary solution for certain conditions or symptoms, in the long run we need to look at the entirety of our inner environment.

The overall environment of the intestines that houses the microbes is what is most important because without a habitable environment for a diverse, helpful microbiome, we may end up with one that's more hostile and simplistic. In terms of digestion, a less than hospitable environment may translate into varying degrees of gas, bloating, distention, pain, cramping, and foul-smelling gas and put us on the Bristol chart more toward number one or number seven, meaning more toward constipation or diarrhea. This is a circumstance in which probiotics may be useful to some extent. Although they don't repopulate the gut, they may play a transient role in improving the gut environment, and they do have the capacity to help alleviate some discomfort on their way through the alimentary canal and out of the body.

Knowing that what we currently have at our disposal are probiotics that don't colonize, some companies are now claiming—and many consumers are hoping—that the supplemental microbes can actually help create a better living environment in the gut. One of the ways this may happen is if the little beings survive long enough to make it into the colon and do some good by helping to kill off less desirable microbes on their way through. This would conceivably free up space for the helpful microbes that already inhabit the gut. Some of the microbes ingested in probiotic supplements are already dead on their way through the gut but contain metabolites that are balancing to the immune system. In fact, many of these microbes are probably dead by the time they get into your body or halfway through it, but they contain helpful substances and may have secreted metabolites that the body can use to its benefit.

The Eastern medicine approach is to work toward cultivating the gut environment through diet and lifestyle modification. What we want is a moist environment with the right amount of mucus; intelligent, balanced immune and inflammatory responses; good enteric (intestinal) neuromuscular communication; and a steady, varied food supply for beneficial inhabitants. We want a Goldilocks gut: not too hot, not too cold, not too wet, not too dry, not too fast, not too slow, but *just right*. Without a good environment to live in, beneficial strains or a diversity of beneficial strains may get crowded out by other less health-promoting critters that take over and disrupt the equilibrium. If out of balance, we need to clean up our diets and habits and retill our inner soil. By providing the proper nutrition and optimizing living conditions for our little helpers we can encourage a beneficial shift in our microbiome. We can clean up our inner neighborhood.

> We want a Goldilocks gut: not too hot, not too cold, not too wet, not too dry, not too fast, not too slow, but *just right*.

Eastern medicine has honored the power of digestion for millennia. It has a repertoire of remedies that help to nudge the body in the right direction so it can take over and maintain balance without the need, in most cases, for lifelong supplementation. It recognizes the body's wisdom and natural impulse to heal. Most of the time we just need to get out of the way and let it do so. Our modern inclination, however, is to randomly try self-prescribed supplements or lean on over-the-counter (OTC) medications.

Probiotics are part of this supplement/OTC craze. They come as capsules, powders, and additives to foods made up of millions or billions of "live" microbes. The species used are chosen based upon studies that show their beneficial effects in the body. Sometimes it's a mouse's body, sometimes human trials are responsible for the findings. Most probiotics are tested as individual strains, not the actual formulation the consumer purchases. There are some exceptions, but usually the product contains species that are linked to studies that show beneficial results. The thing is, a species can have a multitude of individual strains, and each strain can have very different effects. Just as *Homo sapiens* are all individuals, so are the members of the *Lactobacillus* species, for example. Usually the specific strain that's in a supplement is not listed on the label, only the species name is there. And oftentimes the specific strain shown in studies to have a positive effect in the body is not the one in your supplement bottle. When we purchase probiotics, we are trusting that what is in the supplement is the same thing we hear talked about that can help us, and that is not always the case.

Some companies manufacture supplemental probiotics in single strains and others have multiple strains. Some need to be refrigerated and some are labeled as shelf stable. These are live ingredients, so what is keeping them alive at room temperature on a store shelf? If probiotics need to be refrigerated, did they remain refrigerated on their way to the store or to your door? What is the guarantee that they will make it to your fridge without some time in a box on the floor of the natural food store or near the heater of your car on the drive home? What is the guarantee there's enough to eat for the probiotic strains (food for these critters is called prebiotics) to sustain their populations in the supplement? Where's the guarantee they'll survive your stomach acids and enzymes? What if you're just swallowing a billion decomposing microbes, hoping that you will receive all the benefits of not just the dead microbes, but the live ingredients? The claim on the label is a certain number of live microbes, "at the time of manufacture." For those products that are shelf stable, there is a whole other set of variables. Some companies are creating their own proprietary processes for keeping the microbes in hibernation until they make it into the gut. Some are using soil-based microbes that are in spore form. This means that they naturally are in a protective spore, and don't "wake up" until they reach the optimal environment for them to survive in, namely, the colon. Many of these species are less researched, and some have not been proven to be entirely safe. Some of these spore-based microbes may actually be risky for people with certain medical conditions.

Maybe they cost you $50, maybe $15. Whatever the case, there is no guarantee. Not only that, sometimes the strains being consumed are actually not what the person needs. I've seen people experience adverse reactions from taking them. Yet there is a gigantic market for probiotics. People do report they've made a difference with regard to vaginal health or bowel regularity when they take them, but not all notice a difference. What I recommend as a practitioner is that if you don't have any problems, or you're experiencing only mild discomfort, talk about it with your doctor and your holistic practitioner. It is very likely there is something that can be done, dietarily or otherwise, at home for free.

I'm not telling you not to take probiotics, but I do encourage you to have all the facts you can to make an informed decision about your health. We don't actually know what the long-term effects of this kind of supplementation are. It hasn't been studied yet. Eastern medicine *has* been, for thousands of years. Generally speaking, the more bioavailable something is—i.e., naturally occurring and easily digestible—the better nourishment it provides. Products created from scratch in a lab are not considered natural by Eastern standards. People utilizing FMT to cure recurrent C. diff in antibiotic-resistant individuals aren't manufacturing the poop; real humans are providing it. Lab techs are simply screening and cleaning it, but that is not the same as manufacturing a pharmaceutical grade, high potency product. It's possible that pumping ourselves with probiotics may actually inhibit our natural flora in some way—like introducing an invasive species to an alien environment. The other thing is that, in most situations, adding probiotics may just act as a bandage covering a bigger problem, namely, an environmental one.

In so-called blue zones around the world, where people are more likely to live into their nineties and beyond, humans consume naturally fermented products. These products are not sterilized and then pumped with some artificial concoction of microbes, as most modern yogurts are. Who knows what symbiosis exists among the strains and natural metabolites, and in their interspecies relationships, in the naturally occurring medium. We also don't know in what ways numbers in a community and ratios among species in unrefined communities, in such foods as miso and raw yogurt, may make the body healthier. That isn't something that can just be replicated in a clonelike fashion in a lab. It's a natural, organic, unpredictable process with variables governed by the untainted pure environment present in the substrate the colonies inhabit before they enter the body. There is an intelligence present in the natural world that we must respect, yet as a culture we continuously think we know better than it. Maybe we just have control issues. We try to control everything to keep ourselves "clean" or "sterile" when what we are doing is distancing our bodies from their inherent natural intelligence so we can successfully interact with an unsterile world. It's a subtle form of control that may potentially be more damaging than a minor personality annoyance.

To be clear, I'm not against probiotics. I just want people to be correctly informed about their action in the body and know that being on probiotic supplements for a lifetime isn't a solution to the average person's digestive distress or recurrent vaginal infections. The research shows that probiotics can provide benefit for such digestive issues as gas, bloating, irregularity, loose bowels, diarrhea, and constipation. Perhaps they provide relief as they pass through, while a damaged intestinal mucosa or ecosystem recovers from a hit of some kind, perhaps stress or an infection. Maybe they provide some relief to women with yeast infections to take the edge off while the host microbiome recovers and takes over again. These are all wonderful things, but ultimately, in the absence of a serious medical condition, do you really want to be taking probiotics for the rest of your life, or even temporarily, if you don't really need them? Perhaps if the knowledge and discipline is there to replenish one's ecosystem with dietary or lifestyle tweaks, people can put the $50 a month they'd save on another supplement toward organic, whole non-GMO foods—and thereby cultivate their own probiotics.

Biofilms

Beyond the individual critters in our microbiomes, we also need to consider protected microcolonies shielded in substances called *biofilms*— protective sheaths that surround a community of microbes and coat the surface they inhabit with a film. Examples of the biofilms you may harbor are those that can form in arteries or the plaque that forms on teeth.[10]

Biofilms exist in every imaginable environment and can protect our health or harm it. Their surfaces are impervious to many foreign particles or invaders, they feed the microbes they shield, and they are a vehicle of communication. These protective barriers are so strong that they are often impervious to antibiotics, which allows pathogens to linger in the body. This can make it difficult to treat illnesses such as Lyme disease and other chronic infections.

Various cleanses or detox protocols propose that the filmy sheaths some see in the toilet are successfully eliminated "mucoid plaques," aka biofilms. Some of this may indeed be invader biofilm; however, some experts believe most of it is probably coming from the protective mucosal lining in the GI tract, and that removing it may make the epithelial layer more susceptible to penetration and inflammation.

We have both harmful and protective biofilms in the body. Researchers think the immune system secretes a substance into the intestinal lumen, or the inside of the GI tube, that encourages biofilm formation. They believe these biofilms anchor themselves to the epithelial lining somehow and are an added line of defense in protecting from epithelial permeation.[11] In addition, these biofilms may serve to keep harmful bacteria from colonizing the gut.[12] I would encourage anyone undertaking a cleanse that boasts removal of this lining to think twice before doing it. As we are finding scientifically, and as Eastern practitioners have known for millennia, a few days of a radical fast or intestinal purge may actually do more harm than good in the long run. We will discuss a holistic form of cleansing in chapter 8.

Diversity and Disease

Optimal stools are a good indication of gut health, meaning that the environment in the gut is like a Goldilocks gut. They may also indicate that there is a decent mix of microbes present. What constitutes this optimal mix of microbes? Most say it's diversity. Greater diversity in microbiome composition doesn't necessarily mean there are more microbe populations that have very different responsibilities in the body, but that the microbiome as a whole has greater resiliency under stress. Microbiome diversity is a key concept when talking about health. Diversity is considered healthy and a lack of diversity falls into the unhealthy category and is classified as a form of dysbiosis. Dysbiosis is basically an unhealthy or imbalanced microbiome.

One way to support a diverse microbiome is by eating a well-balanced diet full of fiber. To diversify the gut microbiome, many recommend a variety of foods each day, and dozens of different plant-based foods per week—at least thirty to be exact. This includes fruits, vegetables, grains, and legumes. Another recommendation for encouraging diversity includes not omitting any food groups or macromolecules if not medically necessary.

Many of the communities in a diverse gut microbiome do the same things, but some may survive better in the face of a hit to the system than another strain that behaves similarly or produces similar metabolites. Having a variety of these similar strains or species colonized in the gut makes the body as a whole more defensible and resilient in response to stress, infection, or trauma than a body with less microbial diversity. The diversity is like having a good cushion of money in the bank in the event of something unexpected happening. The event may still be stressful and uncomfortable, but at least the cushion is there until you get back on your feet.

Now I'm going to throw a wrench in the optimistic view of a healthy, diverse gut microbiome: what we hold as the gold standard actually may not be that great. Some researchers believe that certain microbes we humans have hosted for millennia are becoming or have become extinct. Modern diet, vaccines, antibiotics in our food and as medicine, pollution, toxins, and lifestyles may actually be contributing to the extinction of species we used to harbor. Sadly, although we are aware of what some of these are, there is no way to replace them. There simply isn't a way to make them recolonize our guts that never had them, or where they no longer exist.[13]

When comparing the modern Westerner's microbiome to those of more traditional or tribal communities, scientists have found ours to be way less diverse. Although we may have the resources and technology to survive longer, those with the greater diversity in hunter-gatherer cultures actually live better than us in the sense that they are pretty much free of chronic, autoimmune, and inflammatory conditions. Researchers see a correlation between this different state of health and the microbial diversity in their guts.

Just what can we do to change this trajectory we are on of microbial extinction and microbiome dysbiosis? We can do our best to use the information we have to intelligently and consistently cultivate the environment in our guts and make it as habitable as possible for the beneficial microbes we hope will keep us healthy. Again, we want that Goldilocks gut wall. If it is too dry, then microbes that flourish in that sort of environment may predominate, the protective mucus lining may suffer and there may be inflammation. Our inner skin, the lining of the intestines, needs a healthy mucus lining, so we need to protect the cells lining the gut wall that produce mucin and feed the lubricant-enhancing species with oils and fats. If metabolism is too fast or hot, then we need to slow and cool the transit time and tract respectively. Whatever medicinals we take or dietary changes we make for the better will inevitably feed the communities that balance the immune response, the enteric nerves, and inflammation. If progress is too slow, and mucus too thick or abundant, maybe we need to scrape the mucosal lining with appropriate herbs and roughage; diversify the population with lighter foods, lots of veggies, and spices that promote movement; and not overeat to further bog down our critters. Keep this in mind: even one meal can change the microbiome, as we will see later in this book.

Indigenous vs. Modern Microbiomes: A Closer Look

When it comes to defining a healthy microbiome, we in the modern Western world are looking to indigenous tribes on the other side of the planet. What we consider a healthy or diverse microbiome is a sad representation of it compared to those of indigenous peoples, to some extent due to the extinction issue mentioned above. Most of our hard science on the human microbiome, even that funded by the Human Microbiome Project, the National Institutes of Health research initiative created to further our understanding, is derived from our meager modern-day representations of what a diverse, rich microbiome is. In fact, in the title of his article in the science journal *The Conversation,* microbiome enthusiast and researcher Jeff Leach calls our modern day microbiota a "disaster zone."[14] He suggests that compared to indigenous peoples, particularly the hunter-gatherer Hadza of Tanzania and the microbiomes of our ancestors, our modern day gut flora composition is "the canary in the coal mine" indicating the devastating state of microbial life on planet Earth.[15] Since decreased or lesser diversity is associated with disease, it is also a good indicator of our overall state of health. Despite all of our modern accoutrements, we are less robust than our indigenous counterparts.

Leach suggests that the lack of diversity in our modern microbiomes is due to a combination of factors, such as a lack of regional diversity and filters that foster separation of species in our environment. Regional pools and human interaction with them aren't as well researched as filters that inhibit such interactions. Those filters include increased C-sections, decreased breastfeeding, too much time indoors, antibiotics we take to kill infectious agents, antibiotics in our food, antimicrobial products, and modern hygiene in general.[16] I would further add foods that are sterilized (for example, milk and almonds) and processed foods, particularly those with added preservatives.

Research shows our modern lifestyle and conveniences may not always be in our best interest. A study published in the journal *Nature* reported greater biodiversity overall in unindustrialized rural communities. More specifically, it compared the microbiome of the foraging Hadza tribe to that of an urban Italian control group and found that the Hadza have higher levels of microbial richness and biodiversity, as well as bacteria that may enhance their ability to digest and extract nutrition from certain plant foods. It is worth noting that the Hadza lifestyle is thought to most closely resemble that of hunter-gatherers.[17]

The massive diversity of microbes housed by the Hadza compared to the modern Westerner results in a relatively nonexistent incidence of metabolic, autoimmune, and chronic inflammatory ailments, but due to the harsh realities of their existence, it doesn't translate into longevity. Generally speaking, the goal would be for us to learn from this data and figure out ways to increase our microbial diversity so that we can not only live better, but also live better longer. The ancients from the East who developed longevity practices, dietary recommendations, and teachings about achieving longevity were surely not talking about living a long decrepit life, but one of relative comfort and ease of movement. They advocated consistent movement, breathing practices, meditation, visualization, herbal remedies, mild fasting, and other tools for well-being. Most of this isn't practical for the average modern-day human with a family and career, but hope should not be lost. Eastern medicine lifestyle recommendations for promoting well-being and longevity are doable for many, even those who feel they are too busy. For most it's just a matter of priorities, beliefs, attachments, and values—all mental constructs that need to change in order to help create the foundation for healthy living.

If you're thinking about a stool test to determine microbiome diversity, I would recommend waiting until we have minimally invasive and more accurate testing reflective of what's actually colonizing the gut. A vast majority of the studies being carried out are using or have used stool culture testing that doesn't measure archaea or fungi. Other studies require a colonoscopy and sampling from different sites along the gut wall. All testing is limited at this point for one reason or another. Even with the promise of an ideal test, we need more information about what's in the stool, what it does, and if it's an adequate reflection of what's colonizing the gut and in what proportion.

What I would recommend is to take heed of the information above and start being mindful of bowel habits. The proof is in the pudding, or the poop in this case. Observe your patterns and alter your diet and lifestyle until it shifts toward a four on the Bristol Stool Chart. We will discuss how to do this in part 2.

4

Making Connections

Recognition of the Mesentery (Mo Yuan) and
Interstitium (San Jiao) as Organs

The lower intestines and the small intestines cause leakages
upon the burning spaces, making them overflow below and
causing water (in the system).

From *The Yellow Emperor's Classic of*
Internal Medicine, translated by Ilza Veith

The quote above translates *san jiao,* or triple warmer, as "burning spaces." It discusses the direct connection between the intestines, which house the gut microbiome, and the rest of the body, and highlights how the water metabolism of the body is influenced by gut function through the connection between the gut and the san jiao. The stool is an excellent reflection of what's happening in each region of the san jiao, which is divided into three sections. Everything in the body is directly connected to the gut and everything else through the san jiao. What comes out of the gut and into the san jiao is first filtered by the mo yuan, or membrane source. This structure is another line of defense that is contiguous with the intestines and helps to filter pathogens—hopefully preventing them from entering the san jiao and general circulation. The quality of the gut wall and health of the microbiome, which affects what gets through it and into the mo yuan and then to the rest of the body, is of utmost importance, as is the environment of the mo yuan.

Mesentery/Mo Yuan/Membrane Source

While I was working on my first book, *Handbook of Chinese Medicine and Ayurveda,* I was getting antsy about writing this one. What made me even more restless was the publication of a "new discovery" in Western medicine in January of 2017 that actually was not new at all. It was an acknowledgment of the existence of something the Chinese have treated for millennia: the mesentery organ. Western science already recognized the mesentery, but before it was promoted to organ status it was perceived as not much more than a discontinuous conglomeration of sheaths in the abdominal cavity that anchored the organs to the trunk wall.

More than an anchor, this fascial sheath is intimately connected to, and continuous with, the intestines. This means that immune cells, once having learned in the intestines what is friend and what is foe, can utilize the mesentery as a sort of central hub—like New York's Grand Central Station—before traveling to other parts of the body. They may do this via the large concentrations of blood and lymph vessels present there. Additionally, anything detrimental to the rest of the body that gets through the intestinal wall can get trapped here to be dealt with by the immune system. The mesentery is considered a major route for cells in transit to other parts of the body. In fact, scientists now speculate that this organ may be a route by which cancer cells metasticize.[1]

According to Dr. J. Calvin Coffey, the Irish scientist who is credited with the "discovery" of the new organ, all of our internal organs develop either within or in contact with the mesentery.[2] I find it interesting that he described it this way because in Chinese theory, the mesentery is called the *mo yuan,* or membrane source. Clearly these descriptions of the mesentery indicate its importance as a source of organ and tissue generation, and prompt questions as to what extent its integrity might affect the other organs and their function, either in utero or later in life. Coffey believes this importance goes beyond initial development. He explains that the signals that travel between the intestines and the rest of the body must pass through the mesentery.[3]

Embryonic Connections

Looking into the embryonic history of the mesentery, it is fascinating to note how much comes from the tissue that generates it, called the *mesoderm*. When you were forming in utero, there were three primary tissues that differentiated into the complex miracle now reading this sentence. One of those, the mesoderm, produced the mesentery and all of the other connective tissues in the body, including the blood, lymph, bones, and cartilage. It was also the source of the cardiac, skeletal, and urogenital systems; blood vessels; and smooth muscle.[4]

Buried Traumas

Many contemporary holistic practitioners work with clients at healing traumas buried deep in the body that may have been experienced during fetal development. Biodynamic craniosacral therapy works with the entirety of a person's being starting with their embryologic development, and a major premise of the widely used Nogier style of auricular acupuncture is that we can positively influence the health and well-being of someone by addressing the imprints left in the tissue from unconscious past events. There are acupuncture point protocols for addressing patterns that manifested during the meso-dermal stage of development. The trauma can be lodged in any of the tissues the mesoderm generates, or in the mesoderm itself.

Perhaps this healing can occur because the mesoderm is still with us, both literally and in altered form. Lodged in bone marrow, blood, muscle, and other places in the body are mesenchymal cells, which are adult stem cells that originated from the mesoderm.[5] Perhaps stimulating an individual's ancient memory with intention and an open mind allows for a sort of resonance, or other type of communication that puts those cells into action, or at least stimulates them for a rebalancing of the disordered tissue or issue.

It's interesting to note that the word *mesentery* comes from the Greek *mesenterion,* or *mesos,* "middle," and *enteron,* or intestine.[6] Not only is it in the middle, it actually pulls the intestines into place during fetal development. The intestines follow it into the position they will live in for the rest of the person's life. When the intestines don't get pulled into position properly during gestation, the potential consequence is "twisted bowel," or volvulus. It may be serious enough to block food and liquid from passing through, or it may never be detected.

Disease Formation

As mentioned above, the mesentery used to be looked at only in terms of its structure and its function of structural support, but researchers now believe it plays a role in disease causation. Inflammatory chemicals responsible for creating systemic inflammation are manufactured in the intestines and mesentery, and mesenteric lymph helps distribute them throughout the body. Inflammation-causing substances, like C-reactive protein, are derived from the visceral fat of the mesentery. This implicates the mesentery as a player in metabolic disorders such as diabetes.[7] Fibrocytes—cells associated with wound healing and tissue repair—migrate through the inflamed mesentery to reach the serosal surface of the intestines, and are elevated in those with many autoimmune diseases, such as scleroderma and Crohn's disease.[8] Crohn's is an inflammatory bowel disease, which causes ulcers that can bore through every layer of intestinal tissue, resulting in a range of symptoms. It can be life threatening if not treated. Some recent research has shown that in Crohn's disease the mesentery may be both a causative factor and a contributor to disease progression.[9]

The mesentery is basically an extension of the digestive tract. A 2018 study described the anatomy of the mesentery thus: "During embryological development, the intestinal endoderm is surrounded by the mesenteric mesoderm. The latter makes cellular and connective tissue contributions to developing intestine. This relationship is retained into the adult as a connective tissue continuity between the mesentery and intestine."[10] This relationship was being investigated in terms of Crohn's disease, but the implications for the development of other illnesses are surely there, as the mesentery is definitely involved in systemic inflammation.[11]

When we talk about the mesentery, we need to talk about the mesenteric lymph. Western science recognizes the mesentery's main functions in terms of the lymphatics it houses, and researchers think it may help white blood cells to travel through the intestines. Another study from 2006 described the mesenteric lymph as "the center of the immune anatomy."[12] That statement certainly indicates the importance of this organ. Scientists are also considering its function in the role of the digestive, vascular, and endocrine systems; as the mesentery and its lymph may be part of a previously unrecognized system in Western medicine.[13] This system also involves the interstitium, which we will get to shortly. It is important to note that mesenteric lymph nodes surround major blood vessels and blood vessel junctions, as other lymph nodes do in other parts of the body. Since we know the mesenteric lymph traps translocating bacteria from the intestines, this indicates to me that harmful substances such as microbes, toxins, and rogue cells can get through the blood vessel walls and, if the lymphatic immune cells don't catch them, they can end up at the other end of the body somewhere, stuck in a joint, a tissue, the bloodstream, or interstitial fluid.

As a structure the mesentery is responsible for pulling into place and anchoring the intestines and internal organs to the trunk walls, yet leaving enough space for peristalsis to occur. It provides a safety net for nerves, blood vessels, and veins to traverse the abdominal cavity without being ruptured by bodily movements. It is also a collection net that captures would-be escapees from the gut and prevents them from entering systemic circulation. This is a high filtration area in the body for monitoring micronutrients, particles, and microbes coming from the intestines, and striking down anything that is not in the body's best interest. The mesenteric lymph is in communication with the intestines and has a special connection with them. It maintains fluid homeostasis and blood pressure by regulating interstitial fluid distribution back into systemic circulation. It is also responsible for transporting nutrient material, and houses many components of the immune system, including dendritic cells. Dendritic cells analyze antigens and activate our immune response accordingly.

Small masses of lymphatic tissue containing B lymphocytes are found in the small intestinal wall. Called "Peyer's patches," they are an initial screening spot for identifying potential allergens or invaders and signaling the immune system to activate. The gut-associated lymphoid tissue (GALT) situated along the mucosal lining of the small intestine also helps the body recognize and defend against incoming pathogens, causing antigen intolerance. This means that proteins on food that should be safe to pass through the intestines are screened and may be reacted to, or may not. But the primary screening and the final pass or fail takes place largely in the mesenteric lymph nodes. It is here that the body decides what is friend or foe and when to activate the immune response, sometimes to itself. If there is confusion here, or a hyperactivity of the immune response, that's when autoimmune or inflammatory conditions may result. This immune connection with the mesentery may prove helpful for the future of immunizations. Interestingly, transcutaneous immunizations are being investigated. These immunizations, which are given through the skin rather than by injection into the bloodstream, are highly effective at creating systemic immunity across mucous membranes, but researchers are unsure of their mechanisms of action. What they do know is that there is a skin-gut cross communication when it comes to immunity that is mediated via the mesenteric lymph nodes.[14] In fact, the lining of the gut can be thought of as an inner skin.

Eastern medicine considers the gut, including all of its associated lymphoid tissue, to be the epicenter and origin for the majority of internal diseases. Weakness here also makes us more susceptible to external pathogens. The causative factors behind most disease can be attributed to incorrect manner of living, or lifestyle errors. These include how we live, as we will discuss in part 2 of this book, what times of day/season/year/life we do certain things, and whether our choices are aligned with our mental and physical inclinations or not. Going against intuition, or disregarding what is known to be true or ideal for our physique and life circumstances can be a primary causative factor for disease manifestation and progression. These are surely factors that influence digestive function and the microbiome. If we go against nature long enough, we can confuse the inherent intelligence of the body, and it may end up working against us. If not corrected, it can move beyond being able to correct itself.

Lingering Pathogens

The mo yuan, or membrane source, of Chinese medicine—what I am equating here to the mesentery—is part of this equation. "The membrane source is the area between the viscera and the trunk wall; it is connected to the muscles externally, and is close to the stomach internally."[15] As an extension of the digestive-immune axis, it has been recognized as a place in the body where pathogens may hide out or linger. They can then be triggered by seasonal shifts or any other stressor, and manifest in chronic conditions. Chinese doctors originally recognized these "lingering pathogens" as externally contracted pathogens that invade but don't immediately cause illness. If the original qi is depleted or there is any kind of deep insufficiency, then the pathogen enters (usually through the nose or mouth), oftentimes bypassing initial screening by the immune system (or wei qi), travels through the gut wall into the mesentery, and hangs out only to reemerge at a later time.

A diagnosis of lingering pathogens, according to the traditional definition, can be quite confusing for practitioners to come to. The person has usually been sick for so long that by the time we see them we are inclined to go with whatever signs and symptoms they are presenting. However, if further questioning reveals that they were sick, got better, then got sick again, or that the current ailment did not start with a fever and chills, then a lingering pathogen may be suspected. It may also be detected by the pulse.

One of the wonderful things about Eastern medicine is that it has adapted to change throughout the centuries. Now lingering pathogens may include not only external pathogens inhaled or ingested in one season that rear their ugly heads in the following season, but everything from chronic Lyme disease and associated coinfections to autoimmune diseases such as Hashimoto's, scleroderma, and irritable bowel disease (IBD). As mentioned above, Western scientists think that understanding the function of the mesentery may help with the treatment of various gastrointestinal, inflammatory, and metabolic disorders.

So how do we treat these pathogens that linger in the mo yuan? There is a base formula in Chinese medicine that has been used for centuries to eradicate lingering pathogens. It was developed by seventeenth-century physician Wu You Ke, who is famous for his treatise on epidemics and their treatment, and who believed that pestilential qi—that is, whatever pathogen was causing the epidemic—could hide out in the mo yuan. Wu You Ke's primary formula for clearing the mo yuan is Da Yuan Yin, meaning "reaching the membrane source drink." It is used to treat diseases primarily of a warm nature, or that turn warm once they enter the body.

I believe the components of this highly aromatic formula are useful not only for directly attacking pathogens but also for unblocking clogged lymph ducts. These clogged or blocked ducts would be considered obstructed by dampness and phlegm. We unclog with aromatic substances like those in this formula, as the formula's stated purpose is to unclog, transform phlegm, and clear heat. We can understand unclogging to be clearing the microcirculation, transforming to be rendering toxins harmless, and clearing heat to be also eliminating toxins and reducing inflammation.

Da Yuan Yin was originally indicated for straightforward, more intense symptoms of a malarial type disorder characterized by alternating fever and chills, chest distension, headache, nausea, vomiting, a tongue exhibiting deep red edges and having a turbid coating, and a rapid, wiry pulse.[16] Like any medicine, Eastern medicine has changed and evolved over time. As a result, many of the formulas in the Chinese pharmacopoeia have been adopted to treat presentations different from those originally intended or documented. This formula may be modified to treat other presentations, and other formulas are used to treat lingering pathogens, or membrane source dysfunction. This also occurs in Western medicine when a pharmaceutical is utilized for its secondary or additional benefits for disease symptoms other than those originally intended.

Chinese Herbs for Epidemics

Da Yuan Yin has been modified by some Chinese medicine doctors on the frontlines in China to treat COVID-19. At certain stages of the disease—classified at the time of writing as a cold damp toxin plague—the strong, warming aromatics contained in the Da Yuan Yin formula are absolutely necessary to help the body cope with the onslaught of systemic, life-threatening fluid buildup. Throughout history the Chinese have been plagued by epidemics. Modern life is no different. Because of the severe diseases they've had to deal with over the centuries, Chinese medicine doctors have had to hone their understanding of the true nature of a pathogen as it presents in a given environment, in a particular season. SARS, also a coronavirus, was a different kind of pathogen than SARS-CoV-2, the virus that causes COVID-19. Therefore it cannot be handled in the same way with the same herbs. Not only will they not be effective, they may actually contribute to making the patient's body a more habitable environment for the pathogen, further weakening the body and potentially increasing complications and decreasing chances of recovery. It should be noted that the formulas administered for this and any other epidemic change almost daily as the disease progresses or regresses. The tongue, pulse, stool, strength, and constitution of the patient is also taken into account when writing formulas. It is not a one-size-fits-all scenario. Preventive remedies are also not one size fits all, as the constitution of the person needs to be taken into account and any factors that may predispose them to being a more optimal host for the virus need to be addressed.

For Chinese medicine practitioners and interested herbalists, the formula ingredients for Da Yuan Yin, or reaching the membrane source drink, are as follows:

Cao guo fructus amomi (tsaoko fruit, related to the ginger family): Transforms turbid fluids and phlegm.[17] This herb dries dampness, warms the middle, disperses cold, dissolves stagnation, and removes phlegm. It aids in alleviating the causes of such signs and symptoms as alternating heat and cold, stifling sensation in the chest, nausea, vomiting, and headache.[18] Cao guo is also useful for cold-damp type diarrhea, spleen and stomach coldness from deficiency, meat-stagnation induced indigestion, and phlegm obstruction in the middle burner.[19]

Hou po cortex/*Magnolia officinalis* (magnolia bark): Moves qi in the middle burner, removes stagnation including that from food, dries dampness, descends the qi, and transforms phlegm turbidity.[20]

Bing lang semen/*Areca catechu* (betel nut): Regulates qi, breaks up accumulations, relieves malarial disorders, promotes bowel movements and urination, helps relieve nausea.[21] Bing lang is also antiparasitic.

Huang Qin Radix/*Scutellaria baicalensis* (skullcap root): Clears heat, dries damp, drains fire, and detoxifies.[22]

Zhi Mu Rhizoma/*Annemarrhena asphodeloides* (anemarrhena rhizome): Clears heat, drains fire, clears heat from the qi level, clears heat from the lungs and stomach, moistens, protects the yin, clears deficiency fire, and quenches thirst. It works with cao guo to regulate alternating cold and heat, harmonizes the interior with the exterior, and treats turbid dampness rising upward. It works with huang qin (Chinese skullcap root) to clear excess lung heat and resolve coughing.[23]

Bai Shao Yao Radix/*Paeonia lactiflora* (white peony root): Nourishes the yin and blood, softens the liver, adjusts the *ying* and *wei*, and works with *gan cao* to alleviate epigastric or flank pain.[24]

Gan Cao Radix/*Glycirrhiza uralensis* (licorice root): Moistens the lungs and clears heat and fire toxicity. Resolves phlegm and stops cough, guides herbs into all the regular channels, and harmonizes the effects of the other herbs.[25]

These herbs would be cooked into a strong drink and consumed several times a day until symptoms were relieved, and no longer. Notice that in its construction the fluids of the body were taken into account, preserved, and generated. The qi is moved and heat is cleared. Turbid dampness is transformed and drained, as is phlegm. In Eastern medicine constitutional dampness and phlegm are usually the result of insufficiency of the original qi and/or the digestive (spleen) qi; overabundance of worry, work, and/or food; incorrect foods for body type, strength, or time of year; overly emotional reactivity and stagnant moods; or incorrect lifestyle. When the body can't keep up with what we're doing to it or putting into it mentally or physically, dampness and/or phlegm may be generated. They can also be generated by an external pathogen. Dampness can travel from the digestive tract into the surrounding tissue and be disseminated to other places in the body, where it can lodge and wreak havoc. If it's in the muscles, this may be experienced as heaviness, or even fibromyalgia-like symptoms. If it lodges in a joint, it manifests as pain or arthritic conditions. If it travels to the brain, usually it is more of a mist, and may result in fogginess, memory issues, irrationality, lack of clarity, or mental disorders. If it manifests in the brain more tangibly, it could express as a dementia-type presentation or in the plaques associated with Alzheimer's disease.

This dampness can also be generated in the tissues and their fluid-filled spaces. Digestion takes place in all of the cells of the body, and if the by-products of that cellular metabolism accumulate without being cleared, then inflammation due to dampness can also result as the ama we touched upon in chapter 2. Anything that is generated by the body or ingested but not properly transformed and/or eliminated, assimilated, or cleared is considered toxic to the system in the long run. Practitioners first try to identify where dampness is located and if it is mixed with another substance, and treat accordingly. Whenever there is dampness there is weakness in the digestion.

Communicating via the Mesentery

In Eastern medicine the body is understood to include a number of microsystems where the entire body is represented. Some practitioners focus on auricular, or ear, acupuncture to treat the entire being. Reflexologists focus on the feet. Korean acupuncturists use hand therapy to treat the entire body. The tongue is also a map of the body, and so is the abdomen. In a form of acupuncture called Fu Zhen, or abdominal acupuncture, the practitioner's primary focus is the abdomen. One of my teachers described it as a turtle on the belly. When looking at the belly, visualize a turtle with its head up by the xiphoid process, which is a small extension of the lower part of the sternum, usually ossified in adult humans. Using this model we may be able to communicate with and affect healing in other parts of the body, perhaps through the sensitivity of the mo yuan/mesentery/membrane source. Since the mesentery plays a role in skin-gut communication in terms of systemic immune response as well as hormonal and digestive function, it seems quite plausible.

Interstitium/San Jiao/
Three Environments

We can't really talk about lymph and the mesentery without also addressing an interesting organ in Chinese medicine, the san jiao, which has a lot in common with the newly discovered interstitium organ in Western medicine.[26] It's the fluid-filled spaces between organs and tissues, lined with connective tissue. Honestly, the holistic bodyworker community worldwide sighed, "Finally!" It had long gone undetected by the modern scientific community because the body has to be alive for this organ to be seen. It wasn't until technology advanced enough for researchers to observe the interstitium in living people that it was able to be identified. Previously, all that was observed were walls of connective tissue lining body cavities, wrapping through muscles and around organs.

Known as the triple burner or triple warmer in Chinese medicine, this "new" organ is considered to be between the layers of the body. I prefer to look at the san jiao as three environments that deal with combustion, or metabolizing of substances.

In the Chinese tradition the organs are classified as being more exterior or interior in relationship to one another. External organs are those more hollow organs, open to the outside world, that serve as passageways. Interior organs are those deep, solid structures you never want to have a pathogen enter, like the kidneys and the heart. There is a hinge between these layers called the *shaoyang,* or three environments' transportation and communication pathway. The shaoyang functions as a plane where external pathogens can be kicked out of the body or hide out and linger indefinitely. It vents heat, meaning it can be accessed to help the body release extra heat—which can be due to a pathogen or to one of the body's processes, such as inflammation—and is useful to treat symptoms involving one half of the body. In acupuncture we needle the san jiao channel simultaneously with the gallbladder channel to assist the body in this heat-releasing process; these two channels are the ones responsible for regulating the shaoyang.

The san jiao as an organ is more a structure "without form," as it's famously known to students of Chinese medicine. It was perhaps considered such because, like modern humans, the ancients couldn't see the entirety of it, which includes the connective tissues, lymphatics, the mo yuan/membrane source, and interstitial and extracellular fluids. They couldn't see it, but they felt it and knew it existed. We can think of it as the space that emerged from the mesoderm in gestation and that remains as the receptacle for the movement of the above-mentioned fluids and defined somewhat by membranous sheaths.

Something I've noticed while researching for this book is that in both Eastern and Western medicine, the same fluid or tissue can have a different name depending on its location. This is true of the lymph, interstitial fluid, and plasma in the blood, as well as cerebrospinal fluid. These are all generated from blood plasma and recirculated back through the blood. Blood is actually a form of connective tissue because it is in matrix form, while plasma is the fluid portion of the blood. So technically, the entire body is bathed in and connected by, cellularly and at larger structure levels, connective tissue and the fluid that lies between and within it.

Lymph is formed by plasma, and contains proteins, immune players, and nutrients that are small enough to squeeze through blood vessel walls into the interstitial space between tissues, body compartments, and cells. It is in this space that substances that pressed through the blood vessel walls can lodge, or where the by-products of cellular metabolism in the tissues can be absorbed back into the blood for elimination through the breath, urine, or feces. It's that stupendously simple. When talking about fluid, if it's in the blood vessel, it's plasma; if it's in the interstitial space, it's interstitial fluid; and if it's in the lymphatic vessels, it's lymph. This magical shapeshifting fluid is our inner reservoir of nourishment. What is in it, whether it is moving as it should, and whether we have enough of it can heal us or harm us. This is why the Eastern concept of the san jiao and the *jin* and *ye* are so important.

Jin Ye

Jin and *ye* are two separate words that when combined refer to all the fluids in the body. The word *jin* denotes light and clear fluids that circulate toward the exterior of the body, such as sweat, saliva, and tears. *Ye* means heavy and thick fluids, such as in the organs, joints, and lining the mucous membranes.

Every fluid in the body and brain is classified as jin or ye in the Chinese tradition. There is a highly sophisticated theory of fluid metabolism that is strongly tied to the san jiao, as one of its primary functions is to facilitate the distribution of nutrition to every cell in the body. In this sense, jin ye is synonymous with the *rasa,* or fluids in Ayurveda. These terms don't matter for the purposes of understanding what I'm talking about—just think *fluids*. The san jiao regulates the fluid pathways, and it circulates qi. What does this mean and what exactly is qi? Simply summarized, it's the energetics, magnetics, ionic charges, and radiation circulated throughout, emitting from, and animating the individual. One theory of an aspect of qi is that it is the electromagnetic impulses that travel along connective tissue pathways. These pathways correlate well with the channel or meridian pathways of acupuncture. Some aspects of qi are aligned with what the ancients knew about qi and the san jiao, as well as what we know today about water being an ideal conductor for electricity.

The san jiao can be divided into three functional regions in the body, which are similar to the *tridosha* locations in Ayurveda. The upper jiao, or seat of *kapha* dosha, extends from the diaphragm up, and its environment is likened to a fog or mist; it is responsible for metabolizing gasses. The middle jiao, or *pitta* dosha area, from about the diaphragm to the navel, is like a froth of bubbles that metabolizes food. The lower jiao, from the navel down to the pelvic area, is the area governed by *vata* dosha. Uniquely connected with the nervous system, it is considered a drainage ditch responsible for metabolizing wastes. The microbiome with its environment in the upper burner is a different ecosystem from that in the middle, which is different from that in the lower portion of the body.

Let me explain further. The name of the san jiao organ can be translated as "three burners." It is also translated as "triple burner," "triple energizer," or "triple warmer." It makes the most sense to me to look at it as the three environments in the body, as previously mentioned, especially because of what we know now about the microbiome. When I read Jason D. Robertson and Dr. Wang Ju-Yi's book, *Applied Channel Theory in Chinese Medicine,* I was happy to find that this was how Dr. Wang perceived it too. For simplicity's sake, I will refer to it as the san jiao. This will make more sense to practitioners and those who resonate with the more mainstream translation that includes the idea of warmth, heat, or cooking. Although I'd like to go beyond the simplistic translation of burner, it does need to be discussed. The word *burner* implies that something is being cooked, heated, or burned, and that there is heat being generated, utilized, and distributed in each of the burners. The three primary regions of the san jiao are distinct ecosystems as well as metabolic combustion centers with specific metabolic responsibilities. The combustion of oxygen is primarily at work in the upper burner. The breakdown of food and fluids happens in the middle burner; and further metabolism of the remainder, as well as the intelligence to separate waste from useful nutrients, water from feces, and the momentum required to push this waste out, takes place in the lower burner.

In addition to distributing nutrients and producing fluids, the san jiao plays a role in heat generation and distribution, maintaining thermogenesis and heat transference. The primary microbial communities in the body can be correlated to the three burners: the upper burner houses the lung microbiota, and the skin is under the jurisdiction of the lungs; the middle burner houses the small intestinal microbiota; and the lower burner the large intestinal microbiota. These microbes produce metabolites that generate heat, so the activity of the microbiome is part of the chemical reactions that produce heat in the body. Heat isn't always associated with inflammation; it is the physiological warmth necessary for survival. There's a reason people say *"cold,* dead body," because without this fundamental heat, we wouldn't be alive.

In addition to chemical reactions, another way heat is generated by the san jiao is through movement—for example, the heart beating or the lungs being moved by the diaphragm. Blood is quick, and the speed and friction of it produce heat. Mast cells—migrant cells in the connective tissue matrix and extracellular fluids—release inflammatory chemicals that generate heat. There is also thermal energy released by cellular respiration as well as by the microbes of the internal ecosystem. In other words, there is a lot of warmth being generated in the san jiao. Warmth in the body and the correct balance of warmth and fluids are vital to our good health, and ultimately, our survival.

The san jiao also functions as an irrigation system; it gets fluid where it needs to be and drains out areas that are too boggy. One function of the lymphatic system is similar to this irrigation concept. The san jiao also helps to regulate blood pressure in that the plasma leaving the blood vessels balances the interstitial fluid moving back into them.

The san jiao is a thoroughfare for the passage of nutrients, heat, fluids, and information. These functions of connector and transporter may be key for modern researchers to better understand translocation of particles, cells, or microbes, and communication of information from one part of the body to another. If we look to the lymph as one transport mechanism, it is interesting to note that lymph nodes are located all over the body. This reflects the necessity of filtration due to the migration of pathogens and accumulation of toxic by-products throughout the body. In Eastern medicine it is widely recognized that pathogenic factors, or anything that is someplace it doesn't belong or in a quantity or quality that isn't contributing to homeostasis, can travel through the tissues and lodge pretty much anywhere. This is clearly evident in cases of chronic Lyme, where there may be symptoms in specific areas that are seemingly unrelated to the site of the original tick bite.

A dynamic *yang* (hollow/spacious) organ, one of the six responsible for transport and temporary holding in the body, the san jiao is actually formless. The yang organs include the urinary bladder, gallbladder, small intestine, large intestine, stomach, pericardium, and san jiao. Without form, the san jiao connects and nourishes everything it touches, without holding onto that nourishment or building up anything that shouldn't be there. The *yin* organs—kidneys, liver, heart, lungs, and spleen—are solid and at a deeper level of the body. More vulnerable to attack or damage, they need protection from the yang organs and immune qi. Yang organs are holding receptacles, at least for a time. For example, the bladder holds urine; the large intestine holds feces; the stomach holds food; the gallbladder holds bile; the small intestine holds enzymes, chyme, and chyle; the san jiao holds fluids. But the san jiao is more of a generator, transporter, bather, and connector. It does hold, but what it is holding is in constant movement, or exchange, and is not clearly visible or obvious. Because of this, it has gained an almost ephemeral status. The ancients knew what it did but couldn't see it.

Accessing the San Jiao with Acupuncture

The san jiao is affected by stimulation of any acupuncture point, particularly those that deal with heat transfer or fluid dynamics. Regarding acupuncture and specific san jiao access points on the body, I think it's possible that the point locations indicated could correlate internally with various valves, lymphatic plexuses, or places that stimulate the secretion of fluids or uninhibit blocked fluid transport. For example, the point stomach 30, *qi chong*, is regarded as the meeting point of the stomach channel with the *chong mai*, or penetrating vessel, and is also the upper point of the sea of water and food. As written in the widely accepted textbook *A Manual of Acupuncture*, "When the sea of water and grain is in excess, there is abdominal fullness, and when it is deficient there is hunger with inability to eat."[27] This point is a connection point between the stomach and chong mai, it transfers excess energy/fluid to the chong mai, which is a storage channel for qi and blood. It can also regulate the qi in the lower jiao, which may be affecting the stomach or causing stomach qi to move in the wrong direction. The lower point of the sea of water and food, stomach 36, *zusanli,* is used by many practitioners to balance stomach acidity and nourish the gut microbiome. There are many references between the san jiao and stomach function, including the one in the quote opening this chapter. We access the chong mai in treatment in order to move qi/vitality and blood from this place to other places in the body that may need it, or to right the flow of qi that's going in the wrong direction.

Stomach 30 is one of the points we can use to clear heat from the stomach.[28] This regulating of heat is one of the primary functions of the san jiao. If microbial dysbiosis is causing excess stomach heat, then this point may help to clear it. Ren 5, *shimen,* is the front gathering point of the the qi of the san jiao. It's used to treat fluid stagnation, urinary issues, diarrhea, pain, distension, and uterine issues.

Bladder 39 is the lower *he-sea* point of the san jiao, where qi gathers as it comes in through the channel's distal opening and dives deeper into the sea of bodily qi. Needling this point can help to harmonize or regulate the san jiao, particularly with functional regard to the lower jiao, in that it can clear water and heat through the bladder. In addition, the bladder meridian that this point is on traverses a huge swath of connective tissue, from the inner corner of the eye, over the head, down the entire back and buttocks, down the back of the legs, and to the outside of the pinky toenail. We can access points on this meridian to create change to this entire pathway. It is interesting that the gallbladder meridian, with which the san jiao meridian is paired, also traverses both the front and back of the body, the yin and the yang aspects, just further to the sides. It begins at the outer corner of the eye and zigzags all over the head and trunk, from front to back, until it traverses the iliotibial, or IT band, which is the tendon that runs down the outer thigh and terminates at the fourth toe. These are the two meridians with the largest surface area of sinew pathways (connective tissue and tendinous sheaths) on the body. Oftentimes we utilize a point on the gallbladder channel, gallbladder 41, *zulinqi,* to regulate the san jiao.

Although the mo yuan and san jiao are not recognized as primary locations for housing our microbial inhabitants, they both play indispensable roles in the function of the microbiome. From protection to communication to travel, they are fundamental to the healthy functioning of the body as a whole. They play roles in the distribution of microbiome end products to yin organs, in nutrient transport, waste excretion, conveyance of beneficial microbes to body sites that need certain strains present to function optimally, and in communication axes between the gut and other organs. These include, but are certainly not limited to, the gut-brain axis, gut-skin axis, and gut-kidney axis.

I love all of these connections. They can help inform researchers as to directions to explore, and help Western medicine practitioners understand Eastern concepts. They also help practitioners to communicate Eastern medicine concepts in ways that seem less alien and are easier for patients to adopt into a personal self-care information bank. Finally, they help Western-based Eastern medicine practitioners like me draw parallels to the material from the perspective of twenty-first-century medicine and culture.

PART 2

Practices for Daily Living

Mind Your Microbiome
The True Meaning of Diet

If you correct your mind, the rest of your life will fall into place.

LAO TZU

The brain and the gut are intimately connected, and both directly affect the mind. This effect can be for better or worse, and is largely governed by the gut microbiome and what it is directly or indirectly saying to the brain. In order to understand this entire dynamic, it's vitally important to discuss the nature of the mind and belief, and for our purposes of modifying the microbiome, how the mind and belief specifically relate to diet and the choices we make about it.

Musings on Diata

The primary reasons we experience inadequate digestion and dysbiotic microbiomes in our guts have a lot to do with what we eat and the way we eat; science has proven this. Eastern medicine views food and lifestyle as medicine. We can take all the medicinals in the world, yet ultimately, to fully heal we need to shift the way we live. Changing the way you live means making your self and what your mind and body need a priority over what society advocates, what is trending, bad habits, cravings, and addictions. It's not just about what we eat but how we live, and what we think and feel on a regular basis. Eastern medicine has emphasized this for thousands of years. To understand diet and lifestyle better, let's broaden our understanding of what "diet" actually is. The word we use in English, *diet,* comes from the Greek *diata,* which translates as "way of living." This concept of diet is much more aligned with that of Eastern medicine than modern Western medicine, even though it is said that the philosophy and practice of concepts related to Greek thinkers are the basis of Western medicine and civilization. Somewhere along the line we lost the essence of what diet is, forgetting that, ideally, the way we live has a fundamental basis in who we are at our core, which isn't governed by fads and isolated incidences in sterile lab environments.

In ancient Greece a specific diet was only prescribed when someone was sick with an ailment. Yet nowadays, in an age of advanced scientific technology and information, we run around in confusion, depriving ourselves of various foods, usually for no good reason. *Diata* (way of living) means living in accordance with natural cycles and tendencies. That includes the way we eat, how much we eat, what we eat, and when we eat various types of food. It also includes eating based on each person's strength of digestion and health condition. Eastern medicine views all that we take in and all that we put out as a part of our diet. This is why Eastern medicine practitioners are generally more apt to recommend meditation, yoga, t'ai chi, qigong, walks in nature, avoiding excess, and mindful living. Taken as a whole, that could be described as self-reflection and self-awareness. These practices help us tune in to what's really going on in our minds and bodies, and they have preestablished frameworks for how to modify, improve, or heal our more subtle mental/emotional or energetic patterns, food-related or otherwise. Consistent self-cultivation practice then sets the stage for how we digest information and emotion, and for our thoughts, decisions, choices, and actions.

The diet of Eastern medicine encompasses everything we are

exposed to: our environment, the people we are surrounded by, what we are drawn to or have an aversion to, what we choose to focus on or put our energy into, what we think, and what we take in, whether by choice or not. This now includes electronic information—whether we ever turn off our cellphone, or can resist picking it up when we see a text has come in—and how much time we devote to media, social media, our families, nature, and ourselves. The modern Eastern medicine practitioner's role includes helping clients to at least be aware of this concept of diata, or diet in the traditional sense, and sometimes to hash it out and provide correct guidance. This is why "lifestyle guidance" is listed in most states within the scope of practice under an acupuncture license for Chinese medicine practitioners. The way Ayurveda is practiced here in the West, lifestyle assessment and guidance is the primary emphasis, and the main reason people seek out practitioners.

Time and time again we are inundated with "new" information about how to properly care for ourselves. It usually takes the form of the latest dietary trend, fad, or food to avoid, and we are whacked around like Ping-Pong balls, not knowing which piece of information is right for us, or not recognizing that some information is best for just some individuals some of the time, and may or may not apply to us at all. How do we know? It's amazing that people in one culture can consume a natural food product with minimal repercussions, yet that same item is demonized as a major causative factor of disease in another. Maybe it's the combination of that food with others that aren't synergistic with it, or that it's not the best food to eat every day, that is a cause for imbalance. Perhaps the way its seeds are processed or the way it's grown, stored, or transported is the problem. It could be that it's consumed in excess or not properly prepared. Maybe it isn't in season and the body knows it, and therefore has limited microbial communities to transform it properly, leading to indigestion or inflammation.

When I was in elementary school, we always had margarine at

our house, because butter was on the bad list in the late 1970s and early '80s. One day a local farmer came into our classroom with fresh churned butter from her cows. We ate it on crackers and it was one of the best things I'd ever tasted—creamy, salty, sweet, and delicious. I can remember how amazing it tasted, and that you could put a dollop on a cracker, which I'd never even thought to do with margarine. It also felt like it was good for me and gave me energy, and became part of my body the instant it went into my mouth. This is how food should feel to us—wholesome, tasteful, and nourishing. Needless to say, after that demonstration I never wanted margarine again.

Then it was eggs that had the bad rap. Luckily my parents never jumped on that bandwagon. Eggs are demonized because they're high in cholesterol. Yet I've known people with high cholesterol who continue to eat eggs but lower their cholesterol by modifying their diet in other ways; or maybe they don't eat eggs but still have high cholesterol. Why eliminate a decent source of vitamin D, in a vitamin D–deficient society, if it's unnecessary? Did you know that one egg yolk has almost as much vitamin D as three ounces of beef or a cup of processed, fortified breakfast cereal?[1] One measly yolk. Yet people have become convinced they're better off with just the whites. Ironically, it's the protein in the whites that is the usual cause of egg sensitivities. Who knows, maybe not eating the yolk with the whites for years makes the whites more difficult to digest.

I was thinking about all this the other day when I got an update from one of the few blogs I follow, *True Ayurveda,* called "D-I-E-T, the Four-Letter Word." The author of the post listed more than a hundred diet and food-related beliefs, fasts, fads, and meal plans that have come and gone, and sometimes come again, over the past few hundred years. An eighteenth-century weight-loss diet advised avoiding swamps, because it had been observed that people living near swamps tended to be more obese. A more recent one included a variation of a high-fat tea consumed in arid mountainous regions that was instead made as a coffee drink with butter or coconut oil for energy and stamina. There are good, solid reasons why people in those regions consume butter tea as a staple in their diets, but those reasons don't apply to the average North American's life. It's just something we think might be good for us because it's been deemed the current panacea.[2] Sometimes these diets get their start not from science or medicine but from an industry that stands to gain financially; for example, the bananas and skim milk diet was backed by the United Fruit Company.[3]

Sometimes scientific studies are done in an environment with few to no variables—i.e., not a human environment—or in a very small population with variables that don't confirm results across the board or rule out future adverse effects. These studies, which oftentimes have one-off results, get latched on to and suddenly that diet or food is deemed by the collective to be either good or bad for everyone at all times. If a doctor writes a book on it, it can end up as a best-selling diet plan, possibly generating a whole industry but creating subclinical imbalances in any number of people. While it's clear that even doctors don't always get the holistic picture, sometimes people who are desperate to lose weight or feel better take the information in a diet plan as gospel.

I'll give you an example. I have a very disciplined client who decided to commit to the latest high-fat and protein, low-carb diet designed to put people into fat-burning mode so they will lose weight. My client was determined to last an entire thirty days on this diet. She began eating bacon every day, resulting in obvious gallbladder dysfunction symptoms. She felt awful but wouldn't eat anything not prescribed by the diet. She continued through the diet, coming in for acupuncture to treat her gallbladder-related complaints. When I suggested, rather graciously, that she cut back on the bacon, she said she wouldn't do that because she was determined to do the entire 30-day plan she committed to.

Sound ridiculous? Well, it is, but I'd venture a guess that we all do similar things at some time or other because of a belief we cling to or a commitment we've made. You can see the power your mind has over your body, for better or worse, if you consider the following. Have you never eaten something your body said no to, or have you never starved yourself (in the modern sense of the word), or have you never not eaten something your body wants because "experts" say you shouldn't? Why do you think you shouldn't? Usually because somewhere along the line someone told you that, and for some reason many of us are wired to abandon our own common sense and sense of self-knowing. See if any of these sound familiar: Raw food is good, but butter, eggs, and salt are bad. Cigarettes are good to tame cravings, ice water is good before meals, and all sugar is bad. White rice, wheat, and beans are bad, as are meat, carbohydrates, grains, cooked food, and dairy. The list includes pretty much everything in existence being good and/or bad for some reason.

This is why I encourage people to look to Eastern medicine teachings with respect to diet, in the diata sense of the word. We absorb so much conflicting information about food that our circuits are jumbled and some of us cannot even listen to our own bodies when we experience subclinical, let alone clinical symptoms. From the Eastern approach, diet would be modified long before subclinical symptoms had a chance to take root, and a way of living laid out, taking into account individual tendencies.

Most of us just don't have all the information we need to make an informed decision about what is healthy for us before an idea is codified by the scientific community, then espoused by mass media. Maybe more information is needed, as well as investigation into who researches the information and how that research is done. Yet we keep falling hook, line and sinker for the newest trend. Every few months something else emerges on the scene. Some people who try it may feel better, often temporarily, for reasons I'll discuss in a bit. Sometimes people do get better, it's just the nudge the body needed, and some stay the same.

In the introductions and conclusions to scientific papers there is often mention of the limitations and boundaries of the study, as well as questions prompted by the research. These questions need to be further explored in order to gain a more complete perspective of the study's results and conclusions, but are rarely mentioned when a study's results are broadcast on the news or social media. We tend to grasp at what we like or hope for about the information, and run with that. We hear about a friend or neighbor who tried this or that and felt great, attributing clear skin or weight loss to the new wonder remedy. Rarely do we examine how that person is similar to or different from us, or what else in their lives may have shifted, been left out, experienced, or introduced near the same time as *x* or *y* diet or protocol. Perhaps the diet or substance was a catalyst that worked to flip a switch in that particular body, but shouldn't be a long-term staple of diet, even for that person. Oftentimes when people decide to make a change, their biology changes with that decision and effort, or they implement many other changes as well, or something changed in their life that caused the shift toward making more life-sustaining choices. We are hopeful, whimsical, and naive about panaceas. In our enthusiasm we can at the least be misguided and waste our time and energy, or at worst do harm to ourselves, all in the name of science and good health, and with the best of intentions.

It is so common to hear people say, "My grandmother did this when I got sick and I always felt better." Or we hear about grandparents who ate this or that every day and lived into their nineties with good quality of life. Yet many of us don't do these things ourselves. It is easier to make choices based upon what is easiest and quickest, what the mass culture believes, or what the latest diet bestseller espouses than what our own family elders have handed down both in dialogue and in practice.

Part of dietary modification is listening to the body and making thoughtful choices. Most people are disconnected from this process and, as a result, don't know where to start and feel that they will fail at it. That belief is the first thing in the diet that needs to be modified. Only when you're listening to your body, as well as thinking clearly without bias, can you make a truly informed decision about what is right for you in any given moment. Thinking *and* feeling need to be taken into account. Feelings aren't just something we're supposed to restrain or express; often they are part of the language of an abandoned body that is crying out for help. Part of this body is the microbiome, constantly sending signals to the brain. We learned from the ancient Greeks to emphasize reason over feeling, but this concept is just one end on the spectrum of how to navigate through life. The other is definitely feeling, which I will include here as a language of the subconscious, unconscious, and superconscious that is utilized by both instinct and intuition. Again, it is tied to the microbiome. Researchers are finding that even decisions made based on intellectual processing involve a good degree of unconscious emotional information being transmitted by the body. As it turns out, most of our decisions are made using a combination of thinking and feeling, even if we don't realize it.

Do you know people who get angry when they get hungry? This is something that is so common that we have the slang *hangry* to describe it. Often associated with pitta dosha in Ayurveda and liver qi stagnation in Chinese medicine, constrained vitality often manifests in anger, even if we don't know why. The gut has been shown to house memories, which were shown in the lab to be stimulated by hunger.[4] The reason for hangry may be that the fierce digestive fluids are disturbing the person's equilibrium, and the body is sending an intense signal to eat so the mucosa doesn't get damaged. That's a perfectly reasonable physiological explanation, but maybe there are highly charged associations or memories in the gut that invoke this emotion. In humans it is not uncommon for anger to actually be a cover for fear. It makes sense that somewhere in the past, that person experienced fear as a result of not being able to eat when hungry, and that fear is coming out as anger. This is something that may even come through the genetic line. An experience from an ancestor may have programmed us to react this way. In the case of any "gut feeling" it is important to feel, acknowledge, and contemplate what the root of it may be. This goes for when we feel hangry, a lack of appetite, a knot, butterflies, or anything else.

Keeping some emotional residue or memory lodged in the gut may have originated as a biological mechanism so that energy wouldn't be lost by having the brain process a lot of incoming stimuli or information. If that's the case, imagine how much our guts are holding on to in this so-called age of information. Whatever the purpose for storing info in the belly, our gut feelings should not be overlooked, as anyone who has one and goes with or against it can attest. Statistics confirm that decisions based solely on intellect prove no more correct than those where gut feelings and intuition are taken into account. Conversely, however, sometimes gut feelings can actually impede good decision-making. When survival isn't at risk, the gut can direct us to focus on the wrong information.[5] Is this a gut feeling based on fear? Where is it coming from? The more self-aware we become, the greater opportunity we have to recognize reactive patterning and shift the dynamic. By cultivating awareness and practicing knowing our intuition, we can avoid being reactive to situations that no longer exist.

It may very well be that the majority of the focus of study on the human microbiome is about the gut because it has an influence on so

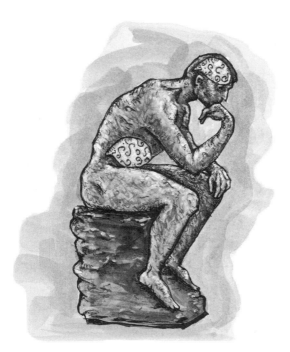

Thinking involves the brain in the head *and* the brain in the belly.

much. It affects everything, actually, including such seemingly intangible physiological processes as those of the mind and emotional states. The mechanisms through which this occurs are still being studied, but there have been some interesting discoveries. I use the term *discovery* loosely because the connection between the mind and the body, particularly the gut, has always been apparent in Eastern medicine, where gut dysfunction plays a recognized role in psychiatric disorders, both directly and indirectly.

Whether the medicine is from the East or West, the mental and emotional puppeteering from the large intestine may manifest from anything as extreme as a clinical diagnosis to something as seemingly innocuous, yet disturbing, as a fleeting sense of vague nervousness or anxiety without definitive cause. Modern science and medicine are finally recognizing the importance of our emotional and mental states on physical health in a way they previously hadn't. This is all thanks to their discoveries pertaining to the gut microbiome.

Everything from simple emotional states to complex syndromes such as autism are being shown to have links to gut function. These mind-gut links are largely being studied in the hope of devising appropriate psychobiotics—pre- and probiotic supplements filled with microbes found to positively influence gut-brain communications in the presence of psychological or brain diseases.[6] Scientists have found that certain syndromes are linked with different states of dysbiosis, but the information they have is in its infancy and it's unclear which came first: the syndrome or the dysbiosis. Regardless, in mouse studies it appears as though they've had relative success in treating mental/emotional symptoms of Alzheimer's, autism, various bacterial infections, diabetes, and postinflammatory anxiety.[7]

In addition to the gut, there are other places in and around the body where microbial communities are in communication with the brain and influence our brain and/or mental state. These include the oral microbiome, which has recently been implicated in Alzheimer's disease, as mentioned earlier in this book; and the aerobiome and exposome, which is the cloud of chemicals and microbes we emit and inhale, that has been shown to affect the mind as well. For example, researchers working on a device that measures the exposome have found that a substance we breathe causes us to feel joy.[8]

Many researchers and doctors have come forward in the past few decades who have recognized the mind-body connection. For example, stem-cell biologist Bruce Lipton produced studies of the connection between mind and body and found that gene expression can be influenced by the mind. His influence popularized a field of study called epigenetics. Current studies go both ways: how the microbiome is affecting our mental and emotional states, and conversely, how emotional states may affect the microbiome.

How Does This All Play Out?

We house a bidirectional communication network called the gut-brain axis, meaning that the gut is directly linked to the brain's cognitive and emotional centers.[9] This axis includes five systems: the autonomic nervous system, the enteric nervous system, the neuroendocrine system, the enteroendocrine system, and the neuroimmune system.[10] The autonomic nervous system includes the brain, spinal cord, and nerves that carry messages to and from the brain, most notably the vagus nerve. The enteric nervous system has as many neurons as the spinal cord and has been called "the second brain."[11] It senses what is in the gut and sends this information to the brain. What it is sensing includes not only the food we eat but our microbial inhabitants, their metabolites, medications, and so on. Since it cannot carry all this information from the gut to the brain on its own, it relies on interaction with the other systems, such as the immune system and the epithelial defense systems. The neuroendocrine system is made up of neurons, glands, tissues, and the substances they produce and receive in order to regulate bodily processes. The enteroendocrine system is a subset of the endocrine system that is made up of endocrine cells present in the GI tract and pancreas. The neuroimmune system protects the neurons from pathogens. Through these routes of the gut-brain axis the gut microbiome can influence not only mood but also neural development, cognition, and behavior.[12]

There is also evidence suggesting that behavior can alter the composition of the microbiome, thereby having an impact on psychological states via the gut-brain axis. Integrating mindfulness practices or meditating, for example, reduces stress and thereby positively impacts the microbiome, creating more positive moods.[13] Diaphragmatic breathing is another positive behavior that influences the gut for the better by massaging the gut-brain axis's central highway, the vagus nerve. When the diaphragm moves up and down it stimulates the parasympathetic nervous system via this nerve, thereby inducing a rest-and-digest state and alleviating stress. Other behaviors have been shown to alter the microbiome in such a way as to potentially create negative mental states. These include excess alcohol consumption, smoking, and disruption of the circadian rhythm.[14] Famous fourteenth-century Chinese doctor Zhu Dan-xi believed that all diseases are caused by depression, and that as long as the qi and blood are kept in harmony and depression prevented, disease cannot take root.

Perhaps behavior can influence the microbiome in such a way as to affect the intestinal secretion of serotonin, thereby influencing gut motility in people who experience chronic constipation. Serotonin produced in the gut does indeed affect gut motility, and any disruption in the process of manufacture can lead to IBS symptoms.[15]

The enteroendocrine system consists of individual cells scattered throughout the intestinal epithelium, which manufacture and secrete hormones. We used to think these cells secreted hormones into the systemic circulation to affect distant organ systems, but this is being called into question by researchers. It's now believed that these cells can communicate directly with the enteric nervous system and influence the physiology this way. Not only that, they are equipped with sensing receptors that monitor their environment. They can not only sense microbes but a vast array of other stimuli: amino acids, carbohydrates, peptides, nutrients, and toxins, to name a few. And get this. Ready for it? They have taste receptors on them! Some enteroendocrine cells in the proximal intestine have bitter taste receptors.[16] More and more we are finding that there are taste receptors in unexpected internal parts of the body.

In Eastern medicine taste is a major determinant of the herbs and foods recommended for various conditions and body types. The tastes affect organs and physiological processes that have an impact on how we behave and feel. In addition to that, certain foods are recognized for their ability to create more mental activity, create a sense of fogginess or stuck thinking, or foster calm and mental clarity. Examples of mental stimulants are raw onions and garlic and caffeine. It is recommended to avoid these things at night as they may make sleep unsettled. Heavy foods, leftovers, and processed foods may all make us feel sluggish mentally. Canned, frozen, and old, dry foods as well as meat and liquor are all dulling to the mind. Fresh, whole foods cooked to perfection with just the right amount of flavor, such as broths, easily digested rice and mung bean dishes, steamed seasonal vegetables, fresh yogurt, raw milk, buttermilk, butter, and ghee will calm the mind. Emotional states affect the neuromuscular action of the gastrointestinal tract, as well as the secretion of acids, bile, and enzymes. For example, fear increases contractions in the large intestine, but decreases them in the stomach and small intestine. Anger increases contractions in the whole tube, and sadness slows them down.

Stress, or rather our lack of tolerance for it, as we have been hearing for decades, has an adverse effect on the body and mind. A Canadian study published in 2016 found that the microbiomes of red squirrels were healthier and more diverse the lower their stress hormones were.[17] In other studies, scientists raised completely sterile mice and introduced various microbes into their systems to see what would happen. They found that lab animals without gut microbiomes had altered brain development in areas responsible for emotional processing.[18] This sounds like the Ayurvedic concept of what happens to humans when the agni, or metabolic fire associated with pitta, in the brain is low. It is known to create mental imbalance and illness.

Not only does the gut microbiome change brain chemistry and behavior, but it can do so without influence from the autonomic nervous system, or GI neurotransmitters.[19] It uses the vagus nerve, neuroimmune pathways, and neuroendocrine pathways as its methods of communication or information transfer. Because of all of this and more, some researchers have suggested renaming the gut-brain axis the microbiome-gut-brain axis.

In twelfth-century China, Li Dong-yuan founded the Earth school of diagnosis and treatment. He believed the spleen and stomach systems—digestion, essentially—to be the foundation for the functioning of the body and defined the primary cause of disease to be a weakened digestive tract. He taught that no pathogen could overcome a person with strong digestive functioning and that the root of even contracting an external pathogen is deficient digestive functioning. Digestive function includes not just evacuation but the intake, breaking down, transformation, assimilation, and transportation of food and fluids throughout the body. Regardless of pathology—that is, what disease and where it is manifesting—the spleen and stomach/digestive function must be tonified, or strengthened. Li Dong-yuan cited intensive overthinking as a primary cause of damage to digestive function. *Pensiveness* is the word used to describe constant mental fixation. It's basically what most of us do on a daily basis. This overthinking directly affects the stomach and the spleen. His amazing text, the *Pi Wei Lun,* or *Treatise on the Spleen and Stomach,* is comprised of remedies for harmonizing the digestive tract.

Chinese medicine has a category of chronic disease called *gu* syndrome. Gu syndrome refers to any chronic parasitic, viral, spirochete, or microbial infection that can hide out, cover itself in biofilm, and potentially make someone feel sick for years. Often people with gu syndrome have been through the gamut of Western medical testing, which often comes back negative. Gu syndrome is unique because it involves an overgrowth of some pathogen that usually affects digestion, and often manifests as mental and emotional imbalances as well.

Modern Chinese medicine doctor Heiner Fruehauf is an expert on gu syndrome and is known for his categorization of Lyme disease and its coinfections. Fruehauf combines herbs to make formulas that release the external invading pathogenic influences, while also tonifying the underlying deficiency that allowed them to take root. He calls the neurological and mental emotional aspects of gu syndrome "brain gu." Someone suffering with brain gu will often have some abdominal discomfort, but will also manifest with fogginess and more serious mental symptoms, as well as musculoskeletal pain. Gu syndrome, he says, is like pouring oil into flour; it is pervasive and binding and can take months to years to treat. The root of it is, in his opinion, disordered eating and a lifestyle that weakens the body's defenses to a degree that is actually worse now than it was when gu syndrome treatments were originally developed.[20]

In China, phlegm misting the mind is a primary diagnosis in cases of mental/emotional imbalances, also known as *shen* disorders. Phlegm comes from imbalanced digestion and can lead to numerous signs, symptoms, and disease classifications including psychosis, depression, bipolar disorder, schizophrenia, and dizziness, to name a few. Phlegm misting the mind means that as a result of some disorder in the digestion/metabolism of an individual, an "insubstantial" phlegm, one that is as elusive as mist or invisible, can enter the channels and circulate throughout the body. This invisible phlegm obstruction can actually impair nutrient, blood, and gas circulation to and through the brain, resulting in impaired sensory activity and dementia-like disorders. This sounds a lot like the concept of ama in Ayurveda, and particles that get out through the digestive tract as a result of leaky gut or Lyme disease and its coinfections, or autoimmune conditions.

In Ayurveda the transformative fire, or agni, that allows us to digest our emotional states so we can process them can be weak, resulting in an inability to properly break down and assimilate our experiences, thoughts, and feelings. This may lead to rumination and imbalanced emotional experience that negatively affects the digestion. This is just what Li Dong-yuan was saying. There are innumerable examples in the theory and history of Eastern medicine of how the mind and body are interconnected.

As I mentioned above, the microbiome is part of this information network between both mind and body and between organ systems. This may also be the case where gut feelings and instincts are concerned. I would guess that a state of dysbiosis would potentially impair the ability to clearly discern one's intuition. Being influenced by overgrowth or products and actions of microbes due to a lack of harmonious balance in the gut can cause us to feel not quite ourselves. It can create a sense of disconnection with oneself and with others, and encourage depressive sensations and anxieties. These are all blocks to sensing intuition. They promote getting stuck in uncomfortable emotional states, and leave us feeling unmotivated in life. Dysbiosis can lead to feeling confused, or getting mixed signals.

It is so important to not only mind the microbiome dietarily, but to also recognize that it isn't just the food we put in that influences it but the type of emotional charge on our thoughts. The gut-brain axis/connection is a two-way street. It is part of Eastern teachings that what our minds generate internally by choice or habit changes our interior as much as what we eat. This includes our beliefs. What we believe fuels our opinions, and those are charged with emotion. Much of what we believe is taught to us by outside sources—such as our society, family, and friends—as we develop. Many of the issues we have related to being healthy and maintaining a healthy ecosystem are directly tied into what is considered normal or accepted by society and our peers, and as an extension of that, how we view ourselves within those expectations/roles/norms. The internal conflict we generate within ourselves can have a devastating impact on the health of the body, including the microbiome. Look at how many disease states are caused at least in part, if not entirely, by stress and our reactions to it. Many are directly reflected through the gut, such as IBS and what many call a nervous stomach. Unfortunately, once a pattern is initiated, it is very difficult to shift.

In a scientific review investigating the connection between stress reduction practices and the health of the microbiome, it was found that the stress response triggers fight-or-flight, which induces system-wide changes to corticotrophin-releasing hormone, which is the main element that drives the body's response to stress, and catecholamine production (for example, dopamine and epinephrine, also known as adrenaline) that can have an adverse impact on the gut microbiome. When fight-or-flight is activated, neurotransmitters produced in the gut are disrupted, affecting the integrity of the gut barrier.[21] When the body is not in a state of fight-or-flight, the microbiome can produce short chain fatty acids (SCFAs) that inhibit inflammation and have anticancer properties (like the butyrate mentioned in chapter 2). The authors of the review concluded that studies investigating the connections between meditation and the microbiome are warranted.[22] This may well happen, but right now it seems most of the research focus is on disease and the microbiome.

Wisdom of the Sages

Since we know the link between the brain and the gut is a two-way street, it makes sense to heed the advice of the sages and ages and incorporate their wisdom into our way of living. This includes following a regular daily schedule, eating in season, self-reflection, balanced sleep and exercise patterns, taking time for quiet contemplation and creativity, practicing presence, and grounding. Much of this is a matter of changing habits that aren't aligned with the natural cycles and rhythms of life on planet Earth. All of these processes will be detailed in the next chapter. Diet is not only about what we're eating, but all that we ingest or take in through the five senses, what we do with that information in our minds, and what we send deeper into the tissues from the brain via the mind's thinking and emotional patterns.

Emotional Expression

Modern science is exploring the concept of memories stored in bodily tissues, which is also a precept of Eastern medicine. Vasant Lad, pre-eminent Ayurvedic doctor and teacher, teaches that traumatic and chronic emotional experiences "crystallize" in the tissue as a form of ama, or toxins. Theoretically these can be cleansed, and the associated emotion may surface as the charged memories arise and are released. The tissues and organs must allow the experience of emotional states to rise like a wave and then pass. It is when they stick around or we get stuck in them, or perhaps continually revisit them, that they become problematic. It is then that the organ system responsible for processing them becomes burdened by the ama and can be damaged, as each organ is tasked with the responsibility to process the molecules associated with allowing us to feel our emotions.

In Chinese medicine the emotional states are associated with organs that each house an aspect of our consciousness. The heart is responsible for processing joy; the lungs, grief; the kidneys, fear; the liver, anger; and the spleen, worry and guilt. In addition to processing these emotional states, the associated organs can be damaged by them if they are in excess or do not merely flow into and out of our awareness, as in the case of stored emotions or recurring patterns. An Eastern medicine practitioner consulting with a client asks questions related to these emotions to determine if there is an emotional imbalance contributing to their complaints or patterns. It helps us to recognize when an organ system may be compromised by a lingering or repetitively visited or experienced emotional state. This allows for a complete perspective on the entirety of the person's signs and symptoms, so we can see the person as a completely embodied being, as opposed to parts and pieces. Beyond this, we can discern how the elements and organs are supporting or disempowering one another in the person's mind and body, and even predict conditions that may arise if the energetics of the person, including their lifestyle, don't shift.

The Five Spirits
Wu Shen in Chinese Medicine

Aspects of consciousness and mental/emotional processes are called "spirits." The *pinyin,* or Chinese name written in the Latin alphabet, is *shen,* translated as "mind" or "consciousness." Imagine that our consciousness is splintered into the body as it materializes. When it does, each piece becomes tethered to an organ. This is why, combined with the fact that tissue can store memory, transplant patients oftentimes experience sensations and other phenomena associated with the donor.

The five spirits are interdependent, therefore a long-term imbalance in one will affect the others. Spirit disorders are closely linked to the health of the body.

Shen (spirit) of the heart

Po (bodily soul) of the lungs

Yi (intellect and conscience) of the spleen

Hun (intangible soul) of the liver

Zhi (will) of the kidneys

The spirits, or aspects of consciousness, are addressed in detail in *Handbook of Chinese Medicine and Ayurveda.*

We can see that diet includes not just what we put in our mouths but also what we expose ourselves to and generate internally. I've often heard these internal creations referred to as our "inner pharmacy." Our intentions, mentations, chronic habituated emotional tendencies, and human cells are manufacturing our inner pharmacy in tandem with our microbiome. Because in the grander sense of the word *diet,* everything we are exposed to—knowingly or not, by choice or not—influences us one way or another, it is imperative that we make optimal choices for ourselves. This includes limiting external triggers and negativities. Are you addicted to politics right now and watching the news? Unhook. It won't mean you aren't contributing to society in a meaningful way if you disconnect from media at a certain time each night or for several days or weeks in an effort to stay sane and healthy. You, your family, and community relationships will be much better off if you're sleeping at night and not feeling fearful, angry, or hostile from what you may have seen on the TV or on your phone before bed.

The brain releases chemicals that cause us to feel the emotional states associated with our thoughts. These are secreted into the body where they affect the cells and microbiome. When we obsess with recurring negative thoughts, we are shooting daggers into ourselves, feeding the feeling and thought pattern so it is reinforced each time it reemerges. Every time we stop that train of thought, take a breath, and open to what is happening right now, in the body, without judgement, we stabilize. Not only that, we create the space and the example for others to witness. Like a yawn, emotional expression is contagious.

Conscious Placement of Objects

Our external environment—our surroundings—greatly influences our internal environment. From the climate to the neighborhood we live in, we are an intimate, inseparable part of the natural and community web. The ancients recognized that the way cities, buildings, landscapes, and homes are laid out has an impact on us. The Chinese address this with *feng shui,* and the Indian tradition with *vaastu.*

I have always been affected by my surroundings. We all are, but some people tend to be more sensitive to what surrounds them, or feel a greater conscious impact from their environment. This isn't bad or good; it just is. In Western astrological terminology I'm a Capricorn, and this aspect of my personality was never addressed in any of the books I consulted as a young teenager in an effort to better understand myself. I did, however, have an aha moment when introduced to Jyotish, or Eastern astrology. According to this system I am actually a Cancer, and one of that sign's primary traits is feeling a potent, almost tangible impact from one's surroundings. Perhaps that's why this next bit of microbiome information fascinated me so much.

Architectural construction influences microbial diversity in an indoor environment. Factors such as size of the rooms, connectedness, frequency of occupation, and ventilation impact the microbial ecosystem of a structure.[23] This makes total sense to anyone interested in or practicing feng shui or vaastu, which take into account directional placement of doorways and windows, sunlight progression, and the presence of water, trees, and hills in structure placement. Practitioners of these artful sciences will enter a space and determine where the front door should be, for example, and if it's placed improperly, what can be done to "remedy" the flaw. This is so that energy, qi, prana, or vitality can flow well throughout the space. I believe that this vital flow contains beneficial microbes.

Feng shui and vaastu emphasize "right" and "wrong" placement of furniture and decorative objects, so, for example, how you angle your bed can contribute to a deep, restful sleep or to restless sleep, strange dreams, and insomnia. There are recommendations for adjusting furniture placement to generate prosperity, or adding objects facing certain ways to assist in maintaining good health. Taking this to the next level is Bhaktivedanta Hospital in Mumbai, India, where integrative medicine is practiced. The building was designed to support health and take advantage of natural resources, so the windows are positioned to utilize crosswinds and create ventilation in the hot summer months. Can you imagine a hospital with open windows? Whereas air conditioners can harbor and recirculate dysbiotic microbes, fresh air draws in beneficial bacteria that can colonize places dysbiotic bacteria may otherwise take hold. It both cools the air and circulates prana, or vital energy. In addition, the design took into account the effect of uplifting artwork on the psyches of the patients; beautiful spiritual paintings hang in the halls and rooms. I toured this facility in 2003, and although it is a hospital, it doesn't feel oppressive. It feels like a comfortable place to relax and heal.

Research is now being done in the West on how to incorporate beneficial bacteria into our indoor environments, including hospitals.

Some believe our indoors should be seeded with devices that harbor colonies of beneficial microbes and their food, the way we might hang an air freshener in a car. Perhaps the principles of feng shui and vaastu can lead to some fascinating insight for today's research into this area, and potentially offer clues as to how it can be done naturally, without forcefully imposing it in an artificial way that may have surprisingly unwanted effects. If you'd like to learn more about research being done on indoor ecosystems and how to optimize them, check out the Home Microbiome Project online.

Negative Charge Is a Positive

We experience negative ions as positive energy. The air is charged with negative ions after a rainstorm, around waterfalls, at ocean beaches, and in the mountains. It is also charged with negative ions when we smudge. Native Americans understood this, as it is used in spiritual gatherings to create a sense of calm and sanctity. Smudging is a process of burning sacred herbs, often antimicrobial sage, to clean the air, the individual exposome, and the environment of impurities. We all know we can smoke out bugs on a visible scale, but that may also be happening on a micro scale when we burn sage and allow its heady fragrance to waft around a person or space.

Forest Bathing

"Forest bathing" is the intentional practice of going into the woods to clear the mind and energy. Although it's considered a Japanese practice, anyone who walks in nature anywhere on the planet is already doing it and can attest to the validity of the experience. The act of the walking is good for us, but it isn't necessary to reap the benefits of being in a natural or greenspace; just being there is therapeutic. These spaces are filled with microbes that may assist in increasing immune function and reducing inflammation in the body. This is called the "old friends" hypothesis and is one theory as to why forest bathing is so effective at helping us heal.[24] Another thought is that the radiating surface

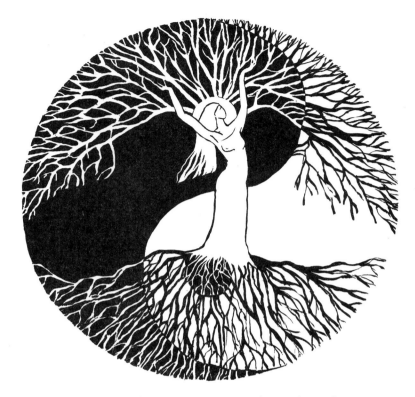

Human vitality is continuous and interdependent
with that of the natural world.

temperature of these areas is cooling to the body, which is linked to positive health benefits.[25]

Just breathing the air in a wooded area or undeveloped greenspace is therapeutic. Trees, fungi, shrubs, and even the forest floor emit terpenes, or chemicals that determine how things smell. Some of these have antitumor, neuroprotective, anti-inflammatory, cortisol regulating, and immune enhancing effects on us. We absorb them through our skin and through our lungs.[26]

In Eastern medicine the forest, trees, greenery, and greenspace are all associated with the liver system. This large organ behind your lower ribs on the right side of your body is responsible for a multitude of physiological processes in both Western and Eastern medicine. In

Eastern medicine it's associated with the elements of wood, space, and air, energetics that allow us to experience sensations of spaciousness in our minds and openness of movement and growth in our bodies. When inhibited, we feel stuck, depressed, anxious, insecure, spacey, unmotivated, and we lack creativity. It is just the opposite experience when we have a smooth flow of liver vitality in our bodies and minds. We feel light, limber, motivated, creative, calm, nourished, and whole.

I am so lucky to be in Saratoga Springs, New York, just a couple of miles from Saratoga Spa State Park. It is a beautiful, underdeveloped treasure trove of streams, wooded trails, mineral springs, mineral baths, and geysers. The combination of all of these natural elements creates an optimal forest bathing experience. The air is bountiful with nourishing, energizing, uplifting qualities. I once overheard the local water guru and natural site guide tell a group about the high lithium content in the air. Just breathing in this park elevates mood, which alters the inner pharmacy for the better. Even in the winter months you can smell the earth and trees. It is easy to ignore the beauty where we live, or not go out into those places regularly. I encourage you to get out and explore nature in your own neck of the woods. Your body, mind, and microbes will thank you for it.

6

Food for Vitalizing Mind and Body

General Guidelines for Health

We are what we repeatedly do; excellence is then not an act, but a habit.

ARISTOTLE

Throughout this book I've mentioned things to be aware of for overall health, including that of our microbiomes. Now it's time to delve more into specifics. I always get questions about what not to eat, what to eat, body-mind type, and how to eat according to constitution. In this chapter I'd like to address some basic, across-the-board dietary recommendations that apply regardless of body-mind type, because each one of us is a unique combination of all the body-mind types, and these practices are the best place to begin. Below is food for thought on food and personal habits surrounding it.

First I'd like to set a new mindset, a new intention as we move forward: Food is not bad. When I use the word *food* I use it in the Eastern medicine context, which is not the broad sense of anything edible but rather, what is nourishing to and vitalizes the mind and body. What is vitalizing varies from person to person and can change within a person at any time of the day, month, or year. Vitalizing food nourishes and

126

cleanses without depleting the system. In Eastern medicine we analyze imbalance based on a deficiency or an excess. Deficiency means there is a lack of vitality in one form or another, in one place or another in the body or mind. It can also mean there is a lack of circulation of vitality to an area. Excess means there is a pathological overabundance of some substance in one form or another in one place or another in the body, which can cause a blockage to circulation of qi (vitality), blood, and fluids.

Vitality and Circulation

Circulation includes all the moving interactions throughout the body. More than just blood circulation, it includes all fluid circulation and the communication among bodily organs, tissues, microbes, and cells. The lymph, interstitial fluid, and cerebrospinal fluid are all part of the system of circulation. The metabolites and chemicals that create an effect in the body need to reach or signal their desired target in order to maintain homeostasis. Essentially, every part of the body needs to talk to every other part at some point, whether directly or indirectly. This communication process takes place via circulation of blood, fluid, nerve impulses, metabolites, proteins, cells, hormones, and forces we are yet to discover under the microscope or through radiological, nuclear, or other imagery. In addition, we emit various kinds of radiation, glow with electromagnetism, and emit microbes. There is not a complete scientific explanation for all the ins and outs of all of these processes.

In Eastern medicine all of this flow or circulation and communication among tissues is governed by vital energy, variously known as qi, prana, or *ki*. For simplicity, I will use the term "vitality." This vitality is present in all of nature and takes many forms. If it is in your gut, it is the vitality of your food. If it is in the plasma, it is the vitality of circulating nutrients; in the skin layer, it is the vitality of the immune defenses, or wei qi. Vitality moves in specific directions along connective tissue pathways. There is a vital force that moves up, one that moves down, one that circulates outward, one inward, one that vitalizes digestion, and one that vitalizes the brain. Vitality is an animating force in general, and is subdivided into forces that govern various bodily and mental functions. Anything that is alive has vitality charging it and keeping it alive.

I believe the ancients recognized this in the microbiome. Because they lacked microscopes, they had to infer from observation, similar to what physicist Niels Bohr did when studying the atom. Since the microbiome is composed of many types of alive entities that serve a multitude of physiological and even emotional purposes in the body, it makes perfect sense that the vitality we receive from food isn't just the food, but what microbes come in with it and what the microbiome does with it. There isn't just some ethereal vitality to the immune system; there's an exchange of information and an intelligence within the microbiome and the human cells of the body that allows them to interact, teach, and learn. It isn't just nutrients from food that are distributed to all the cells but nutrition that is derived from the microbes within us. And there isn't just vital digestive capacity but an interplay of many parts, including the microbiome, that combine to allow for breakdown and assimilation of nutrients. There is even a form of vitality that stays on with the body after death. This may, in fact, be due to beneficial communities within the microbiome that preserve the tissue; a more tangible aspect of vitality that persists when the soul or animating essence leaves, continuing to live when our primary consciousness is gone.

Circulation includes the most minute microcirculation in the tissues as well as the large-scale general circulation. It includes plasma, blood, vitality, fluids, nutrition, immunity, essence, spirit, and consciousness. Any interruption to the flow of any of this circulation to any place in the body causes imbalance that results in excess or deficiency. The ancients recognized this and created bodywork techniques and medicinal herbal protocols to be smoked, ingested, applied, or administered rectally or vaginally to liberate all movement in the body and mind.

How well the circulation works is largely dependent on our movement, the quality of the breath, and, as mentioned in the previous chapter, our diets and our digestion—in the typical sense of the words and in the sense of lifestyle and emotional processing.

One Size Fits All, or Does It?

There is no single diet or eating plan that is best for all people all the time, or even for one person all the time or all people some of the time.

Eastern medicine offers elaborate dietary and lifestyle guidelines based upon how the person is presenting, taking into account their excesses and deficiencies. The food guidelines are organized according to whether a substance has a heating or cooling effect on the body, an anabolic or catabolic effect, and a food's taste. The tastes are known to have distinct effects on tissues and organs, the mind, and the being as a whole. Foods are categorized into groups based on the taste and the thermogenic effect on the body that encourage the growth or depletion of any number of substances or processes. I would love to see research into which microorganisms thrive on what tastes, and vice versa. A good basic rule of thumb is to have each of the tastes in every meal (see the box on the following page).

Sometimes people ask me to tell them what they are "supposed" to be eating, and I do this to some extent. But what happens when the advice I give someone about specific foods for the next couple of weeks is held onto indefinitely? I can't guarantee the client will come back for updated recommendations. It is not so simple as one diet list, one consult, one medicinal. Even in Western medicine, stabilization and healing are a process. How many medications will a person with depression, high cholesterol, or high blood pressure cycle through in the course of a few months or decades? How many times have cholesterol or blood pressure meds needed to be changed because the person is intolerant of the first one or two? And what about developing sensitivities or allergic reactions to things you used to be able to take? When these things

Incorporating Each of the Tastes
of Eastern Medicine

In Eastern medicine, foods are categorized by taste as follows: sweet, salty, sour, bitter, pungent, and in Ayurveda, astringent. Astringency may be seen as sort of a subcategory of sour. Chinese medicine also has a bland category. This means a substance has only a subtle taste, with the quality of purity; it may be seen as a subcategory of sweet without having the cloying effects of most sweet foods. Eating a combination of the five primary tastes creates a balanced taste profile entering the body and sidesteps a habitual tendency toward one or two tastes that will eventually lead to imbalance. It may also be a primary factor in creating and maintaining a balanced microbiome. It may seem difficult to some of you reading this right now to incorporate this principle, so I recommend starting by doing it for one meal a day. Then you can work the habit into every meal over time.

Here are examples of foods for each of the five primary tastes and the two subcategories of astringent and bland.

- **Sweet:** Most foods have some element of sweet to them. Examples include whole grains, meats, sweet potatoes, cooked onions, carrots, corn, fruit, sugar, and squashes.
- **Salty:** Salty foods include salt, of course, as well as seaweeds and miso.
- **Sour:** These are vinegars, fermented foods, limes, and lemons.
- **Bitter:** Dandelion greens, collards, kale, parsley, coffee, and arugula.
- **Pungent:** Garlic, raw onion, scallion, radish, chilies.
- **Astringent (Ayurveda):** Pomegranate, beans (considered sweet in Chinese medicine), broccoli, cauliflower, dill, parsley.
- **Bland (Chinese):** Often combined with another taste, examples of foods that are at least partially bland are coix seeds and cucumbers.

It is common for one food to have more than one taste, so different traditions and sources may have slightly different categorizations.

happen, patients usually follow through with the doctor. However, when people ask about their mind-body type or what foods to eat, they may follow through, but only for a time. I think this is because they think their presentation is static, although I always emphasize its shifting nature.

It is difficult work to change your diet. And it is difficult work to understand yourself enough to know which mind-body type is dominant in you at the moment, regardless of your baseline. It takes time, diligence, learning on your own, self-reflection, and objective self-awareness to make sense of it and stick to it. "Knowing" one's type still doesn't solve life. We all need help sometimes, and we all need to pay heed to our own inner guidance.

What's My Type?

Each of us has an original constitution—a baseline type, or *prakruti*—that can be equated to a personal genetic profile. We also have an acquired type, or *vikruti,* which is how our constitution is currently presenting. Both can be assessed by an Ayurveda practitioner through pulse diagnosis. We also have an elemental type that can be assessed by a practitioner skilled in Chinese medicine's five element theory. We all are a combination of all the types, regardless of system, as we all require the requisite foundational elements to be alive. It's a matter of the exact mixture and proportions of elements and qualities, and how we manifest as a result, that makes us all unique. Every snowflake is made of water, but all are different. It is the same with our genetics and with the microbiome. It takes consistency, patience, change, and time to create good lifestyle habits, regardless of mind-body type. I know of an Eastern medicine practitioner who doesn't like to give people their original constitutional assessment the first time he sees them. Here's why.

For most people, knowing what our mind-body type is can offer a tool to make better choices for one's self, as well as reassurance, validation, acceptance of self and others, and a sense of belonging in one's own skin. On the flip side, it may not pertain on a daily basis throughout one's life, it can be used as an excuse for why we do or don't behave certain ways, and can be a limitation. It can make people feel like they've been placed in a box and have the psychological impact of inhibiting growth and change. It can help to heal, but the information can also harm. I have been to a number of courses (and done it myself) where we talk about a personal trait and say, for example, "Oh that's my vata!" Pittas (transformers) tend to proudly boast about their constitution while kaphas (sustainers) are often quietly disappointed by theirs. And vatas can go either way. I once saw a young boy have a meltdown after his pulse was read in a class because he didn't like the practitioner's conclusion; it confirmed for him the things he liked least about himself.

Mind-body constitutional diagnosis doesn't help if the practitioner gets it wrong or your ego has an expectation that gets met (or doesn't). For many people, knowing one's base or primary constitution isn't enough. In terms of acquired constitution, which is the constitution we will focus on here—and the one that needs to be addressed in order to create balance—it is always moving, shifting, dynamic. We must then be honest with what's dominant in any given moment and act accordingly. For example, it's not about eating a pitta-balancing diet because someone says your constitution is primarily pitta (to simplify, hot) or you took an online quiz. It's about having an embodied knowledge of what pitta, heat, or transformation actually is—what it feels like inside your skin, or on it, and what the signs and symptoms of out-of-balance heat in your system are like. Then, it's about knowing when your hot nature is in balance and something else is not, and knowing what to do to rebalance your mind-body factors. If that isn't enough, then we actually need to follow through on that knowledge with action and consistency to effect change. Doing this takes a commitment not only to learn about Eastern mind-body diagnosis and types but also to learning more about yourself. For those who are interested in learning more, constitution is covered in great detail in my book *Handbook of Chinese Medicine and Ayurveda*.

There is also a great deal of interest in microbial constitution. Like genetic testing for determining ancestry, new companies are popping up that test the microbial inhabitants of the gut through a stool sample. They then issue a report stating which microbes were found associated with various diseases, but this is, again, based upon limited knowledge. It can be a good guideline, but it isn't a guarantee the disease process will ever manifest. Remember, we all have staph, for example, but that doesn't mean we all will end up with a life-threatening staph infection one day. This limited information can be problematic for people who are unable to take in such information without allowing it to adversely affect them. I defer to the Risks and Considerations listed on the website of Psomagen, a microbiome testing company.

> You should not assume that any information we may be able to provide to you will be welcome or positive. . . . This information may evoke strong emotions and has the potential to alter your life and worldview. You may discover things about yourself that you may not have the ability to control or change. . . . You may want to consult a lawyer to understand the extent of legal protection of your genetic and microbiome information.[1]

That kind of strong language stopped me in my tracks, because it's so true. It is undeniably the most responsible thing I've ever read in any terms and conditions. It goes on to state the limited scientific research results are founded upon, and the vast wealth of information still to be determined.[2] I wonder, though, how many people read that part? How much easier it is to make assumptions given pieces of information, and then develop worry or anxiety about the results. It is natural to jump to conclusions. It is also potentially damaging, which is why I recommend people read the entire terms and conditions if they decide to test any aspect of the microbiome. It could be that one day the insurance industry starts using it in determining benefits. As an extension of this topic, the Genetic Information Nondiscrimination Act of 2008 (GINA) protects most people from having employers or insurance companies discriminate against them based upon their genetic test results, but not all.[3] I recommend taking a look at this law to know whether or not you are protected by this act, which someday may or may not include genetic information on the microbiome. What is being tested is the genetic information in the poop samples that identify the species in the large intestine. We also need to understand that this is a simple test that only shows some things and not others, and may not accurately reflect the species or strains that actually colonize the gut in great numbers.

Because we are in our infancy in understanding the whole picture pertaining to the microbiome, I feel it is best to implement optimal self-care with regard to our overall health, which inevitably impacts our microbiome. Let's just go back to basics. The scientific information we may glean from studies that have been done is a step in the direction of better understanding overall, but it is far from comprehensive.

We don't have pre- or probiotic, individually tailored, colonizing cocktails to balance mood, signs, symptoms, or diseases, but we have it in our power to do the best we can with the information we do have. This is a combination of scientific information that points to a course of action, our own inherent instincts and intuition, our ability to be more self-aware, and our ability to make decisions that best serve us. This information is based on correct perception of our own experiences along with the wisdom of our elders, ancestors, and human community as a whole.

What to Avoid and What to Eat

One primary tenet of the Eastern medicine traditions is doing what we know in our core is best for us, as opposed to going against it. In Ayurveda, the greatest mistake we can make for ourselves is knowing what is best for us and not doing it. From these traditions, fresh, unmodified foods that are local, seasonal, and free of pesticides and preservatives and fillers are recommended. Just start there. Don't worry if it is "right" for your mind-body type or not. Just start with fresh, local, and as seasonal as possible. Begin a habit of incorporating a trip to the local farmer's market each week, or if it's on winter hiatus, head first for the organic produce section when you go to the market. This simple act will begin to shift eating dynamics. Be honest about the enthusiasm or resistance that arises with this initial recommendation on the path to microbiome well-being. Nurturing the microbiome is also nurturing yourself. A true path to healing involves determination, honesty, will, consistency, allowing, and letting go.

I would secondarily recommend avoiding the following products, or at least limiting them as much as possible: refined sugar; factory-farmed meat; anything processed, boxed, or canned; excessive dairy; yogurt as a food group or meal replacement; processed oils; and refined white flour. If you want to avoid gluten, avoid gluten, but resist regular consumption of gluten-free fake gluten products. Likewise, vegetarian nonmeat products usually have a ton of ingredients in them and are considered another form of processed food, as are lactose-free milk replacements and processed nut milks. As for nut milk, you can make your own with just a few minutes of prep, and it is so wholesome and delicious with no additives.

Have caffeine and alcohol in moderation. And if a restrictive diet isn't medically necessary, avoid that too. The average person can figure out what helps and what harms, and barring some health issue, lose weight without suffering unnecessarily and imbalancing the gut microbiome. You can begin to do this by implementing the recommendations here and in the following chapter.

Minimize Refined Sugar

Between 2018 and 2019, Americans consumed about 11 million metric tons of sugar. If you read labels, it's difficult to find something without sugar added to it, or eat at a restaurant that doesn't add sugar when preparing food. Excessive sugar, particularly refined white sugar, is a cause of imbalance in the body and a major cause of inflammation. Could it be that we are unknowingly desensitizing our taste buds, and consequently our minds, to sweet? It seems we are continually hammering the pancreas, messing with energy levels and moods, and setting ourselves up for metabolic disharmony.

Everyone I've led through a dietary reset cleanse, even without totally eliminating sweet from the diet, has commented on how much it increased sensitivity to sweet taste. Anyone I've ever spoken with who has totally cut out sugar for a short time has said that when it was reintroduced, it was like a flavor explosion. They all also commented that after the first few days of the body getting used to not eating sugar, their energy patterns throughout the day stabilized, there was more inclination to listen to themselves when they'd had enough, and they were more inclined to rest or relax. I have had the experiential realization of what an assault it is to the pancreas to be whipped into action to accommodate the ingestion of something very sweet, such as a commercial piece of candy or even a mass-produced chai. I feel that it's actually a form of subtle violence to do that to the body over and over again. And with sugar in everything from store-bought pasta sauce, to pasta, to ketchup, to pretty much everything, we are operating at a consistent level of sugar intake so our baseline is really high. Actually, like any substance that we can become dependent upon, our tolerance goes up and sweet becomes something we crave more and more. It is a pretty serious problem, as insulin resistance rates and diabetes statistics clearly show.

If you take sugar out of your life for two weeks—including refined white flour, which is metabolized like sugar and acquires a gluelike texture—you may at first feel like you are coming down with the flu for a couple of days. The body aches and fatigue may be intense. Then once that passes, energy levels stabilize and cravings for sugar decrease. When you go back to sugar, make an effort to consume whole food sugars: whole pieces of fruit, honey, and maple syrup. It's also a good idea to moderate the white potatoes, and when you do have them, eat the skin. Use raw honey, because heating it denatures its proteins and lessens its antimicrobial effects. I also like a good maple syrup, again in moderation. If you are going to use sugar, use organic, whole, unrefined cane sugar. Some people also like agave syrup and coconut sugar. Sugar, the way the average person in the United States consumes it, causes dampness and eventually heat in the system. This makes for a sticky substance that can be a food source or haven for pathogens and rogue cells anywhere in the body. It may also obstruct the flow of nutrients and toxins, which equates to absorption and elimination issues at the micro level, and cause issues with microcommunication in the system. Sweet is one of the primary tastes in Eastern medicine nutrition and should not be permanently eliminated entirely. That would be next to impossible in any event, since, as I mentioned already, most foods have an element of sweet to them. I just suggest eliminating unnecessary sugar for a short time to hit the reset button in your body and mind, and allow for a true sense of sweet in your life.

Good Salt Is Critical

In Eastern medicine salt isn't public enemy number one. In fact, adequate amounts of good, mineral-rich salts need to be consumed in order to preserve the mineral balance in the body. In the West we tend to get too much non-mineral-rich salt because what's being consumed most often is harsh white salt, which is overabundantly added to canned, processed, and restaurant-prepared foods. In addition, modern Western society promotes heavy water consumption. This isn't a bad thing, it's just that we may be flushing minerals right out of our tissues and bogging down the interstitium/san jiao. We could be waterlogging ourselves at a more subtle level that has accelerated natural depletion consequences. I believe that this water excess in the absence of adequate nutrition promotes a state of dryness and yin deficiency. Yin deficiency means there is a lack of refreshing coolness to balance heat, and a lack of moisture, juiciness, fluidity, nutritive fluid, lubrication, or lubricant-producing substances in the body. Someone who is yin deficient can present with symptoms like insomnia, agitation, restlessness, irritation, hot flashes, night sweats, inflammation, and dry skin, hair, nails, and membranes. This would equate to an imbalance in *rasa,* or plasma in Ayurveda. I have avoided having to give herbs to some yin deficient clients by recommending they switch to mineral-rich salts, such as Himalayan black or pink salt, and supplement with trace minerals, and these simple tweaks alone have improved many long-standing complaints.

People often ask about lemon water. Lemon is great provided it isn't the only water being consumed, and that there aren't certain liver/stomach disharmonies, such as particular kinds of acidity imbalances. It doesn't contain the entire gamut of minerals, however, and many of us remain depleted. Some people supplement with sugar-free electrolyte supplements or homemade super-diluted Himalayan salt water, also known as Ayurvedic energizing water, but it is preferable to get those minerals from foods most of the time and use supplements only as needed.

Eat More Fiber

We previously discussed fiber and one of the end products of its consumption, butyrate, but it merits further discussion. Not only is it recommended by Erica and Justin Sonnenberg, pioneers in human gut microbiome research and authors of *The Good Gut,* but it's been recognized for thousands of years in Eastern medicine to have a positive impact on the overall well-being of the individual, and for precisely many of the reasons listed here. Fiber scrapes the intestinal walls of excess, adds bulk, can slow hypermetabolic transit time, can speed slow transit, can absorb particles and toxins, and feeds gut microbes that in turn produce metabolites, hormones, and vitamins we need to be healthy. By adding pulses (beans, lentils, and peas) and more veggies to the diet, we are able to accomplish all of this successfully with minimal sacrifice and effort. To scrape the gunk from our insides, we can add insoluble fibers, such as dark leafy greens, celery, and the supplemental antioxidant formula triphala (which we'll discuss further in chapter 8). To add bulk, increase transit time, and optimize fermentation by microbes in the large intestine, increase intake of soluble fiber. Sources include oatmeal, psyllium, blueberries, nuts, and apples. To feed the good guys in the gut, eat resistant starch such as recooked potatoes, rice, green bananas, legumes, and oats. Many foods contain a combination of both types of fiber, so eat whole fruits and veggies as much as possible, including the skins.

Processed Oils and Other Sketchy Edibles

I am not an angel when it comes to food. I crave things and I often eat them, I clean up my diet and I slack on it at times. Life is busy, hectic, and sometimes traumatic or emotionally taxing. For all these reasons, pretty much all of us slack now and again and eat things we know aren't the best for us, or don't eat enough, or eat too much. I'm with you on that. But there are some things I truly do my best to avoid.

There may not be scientific studies to back up all the anecdotes I share, but there don't need to be. Observation was the science of the past, and although modern science is supposed to be objective, observation is also an aspect of modern scientific theory. Subjective observation may not be scientifically conclusive using the scientific method, but when you hear these stories over and over again, do the research, and try it for yourself with similar results, why would you wait for a scientific study to implement what your body already knows? We all have a personal inner physician constantly whispering to us, and we need to value this information.

Those whispers got very loud for me when Olestra, marketed as a calorie- and cholesterol-free fat substitute, was released back in the 1990s. Produced by synthesizing sugar and vegetable oil, it managed to get approved by the FDA and was used in a variety of food products. It had some success, marketed as Olean, but went out of vogue when it was found to inhibit absorption of certain nutrients and cause unpleasant side effects such as abdominal pain, loose bowel movements, and diarrhea. I recall the first time I ever tried it. My friend was trying to lose weight and was eating Olean chips like it was his job. I tasted one and felt a coating stick to my tongue. Then, as so many of us do, I ignored it and had more. I hadn't been eating fried food at all for a period of time prior to this, which probably made me more aware of this thick greasiness. Although I ate only a handful of those chips, I experienced what felt like a thick film coating my tongue, and as far as I could feel down my throat. I remember thinking that it was going to take some time for my body to cut through that. It felt like I had eaten a viscous wax.

Olean/Olestra is banned in the European Union and Canada but is still legal in the United States. According to Wikipedia, Olean/Olestra has an alternative use under the name "sofra." It is a primary component in deck stain and a power tool lubricant.[4]

Other products we are normally subjected to, knowingly or not, that are banned in other countries include various chemicals in cosmetic and food products. One of these is the use of hormones in livestock. Shown to cause birth defects, they were banned by the European Commission in 1981.[5] Also banned in the E.U. but still used in the U.S. are food dyes that are linked to allergies, hyperactivity in children, and cancer risk: red 40, and yellows 5 and 6.[6]

Brominated vegetable oil (BVO) is banned in Europe and Japan; derived from vegetable oil, it is added to soft drinks to retain the citrus flavor.[7] Azodicarbonamide (ADA), used in commercial breads and yoga mats alike, can be found on the FDA's website despite having been shown to cause tumor growth in female mice. The FDA supports its approval for use based upon the rationale that it was not shown to cause tumor growth in male mice, or in either gender of rat. Also, since it was supplied in such massive quantities that "far exceed estimates" of what a person would consume, the FDA doesn't consider it a risk.[8] I find this to be absolutely ridiculous. First, safety shouldn't be based only on affected gender; second, what study *doesn't* poison animals with ridiculously high dosages of substances in an effort to determine human safety? This is one very clear example of why people need correct, complete information, and to think freely and feel for themselves and honor those thoughts and feelings.

Among the things I really try to avoid are canola oil and other vegetable oils. Used almost everywhere and touted as healthy, I believe they are simply not a good choice. During a dietary reset I led, one client commented that she had eaten out only once, at a charity function. Although she stuck to what she had chosen to eat during her personalized dietary reset, the oil the vegetables were cooked in was the only variable she could track that would account for her resulting discomfort. Prior to that she had been using only a very high-quality olive oil or ghee in her food preparation.

Canola oil and other processed pseudohealthy oils go rancid easily, often during processing. Most vegetable oils, such as corn, soybean, and canola, are deodorized, ostensibly to create a bland taste but perhaps also to eliminate any rancid odor. This process leads to the production of harmful trans fats, and rancid oils overall contribute to free radical increase in the body. They also don't contain the correct balance of omega 3s to 6s, which we know is not optimal for enzyme activity in the body and has an adverse impact on immune functions.[9] We know that high omega 3 diets, of which canola and other processed vegetable oils are *not* a part, increase diversity of the gut microbiome, and that diversity is linked to greater health.[10]

Canola oil has a questionable history. In an article entitled, "Canola Oil Proven to Destroy Your Body and Mind," Joseph Mercola, D.O., talks about its origin. It is common knowledge that canola oil was created from rapeseed, which, in its natural state, is not suitable for human consumption. It began as a crop grown in Canada and was used as motor lubricant during WWII.[11] It was then genetically modified for pest resistance and to increase crop yield, crossbred to significantly reduce glucosinolates and erucic acid (believed to be toxic in high doses), and is now one of Canada's biggest crops. In this same article Dr. Mercola notes that canola oil decreases production of a protein that protects the brain against neuronal damage and cognitive impairment.[12] In a study he cites, mice bred to develop Alzheimer's disease were all fed the same diet except that one group was given canola oil and the other, olive oil. The mice in the olive oil group not only gained less weight, but developed less plaque in their brains.[13]

Why am I so hung up on canola and processed vegetable oils? Not because I want to put Canada's agricultural market into bankruptcy, but because of the fact that so many people have been told they are healthy. In fact, they're harmful for us to consume on a regular basis, even cold-pressed. I encourage people to choose oils that nature produces with little interference from us, like high-quality extra virgin olive oil. Another option is ghee made properly from the milk of grass-fed cows. There are plenty of studies showing the health benefits of these and other natural choices.

Our Broken Connection to the Natural World

You can read anything from anyone these days and find highly opinionated, scientifically validated information on either side of any fence. This is one reason why people are so confused about what to eat. This applies specifically to those of us in industrialized nations who no longer live in harmony with the natural world, but doesn't even begin to take into account the people worldwide being poisoned with artificial diets and limited access to healthy foods for a variety of reasons. Being confused is a kind of luxury when taking the bigger picture into account, but that confusion leads to complications, such as a lack of microbial diversity in the gut, human gut microbe extinction, and totally allowing our food supply to be messed with and messed up because of lack of truth, free thought, common sense, and clarity.

It may not seem as if little extra bits here and there of processed oils, additives, and overindulgences make that much difference. It's true that it's probably not going to hurt the average healthy adult long-term to have some vegetable oil now and again, for example. But the problem lies in the cumulative effect of our exposure. It is consistent consumption that usually creates an imbalance in the subtle functioning of the body. This imbalance can also cause greater sensitivity to small amounts of these and other substances that we wouldn't ordinarily have a problem digesting. In Eastern medicine nothing processed is advised for consumption, and certainly not on a regular basis. Yet the majority of products in the supermarkets most of us have access to is somehow genetically or otherwise modified or processed. GMOs and food additives abound, including at least half a dozen that are banned in Europe. Many of us consume them daily and feed them to our children at home and in our schools. We don't yet know the long-term consequences to this. What we do know is that there is an unprecedented rise in chronic childhood maladies such as asthma, seasonal allergies, peanut allergies, and autism spectrum disorders.

I was born in 1973 and when I went to school it was the rare kid who had a food allergy. EpiPens, now in common usage, weren't available until I was almost through high school. The generation before didn't grow up conscious of peanuts being something that could cause an allergic response. Now you can't send baked goods to preschool with your kid because you might accidentally kill someone, or send another student into anaphylactic shock. This is a very serious problem that isn't showing any signs of slowing. Some theories are that food allergies are caused by high levels of certain pesticides, or that protection from germs and our obsession with antibacterial soap may be the culprits, but whatever the case, we need to get serious about what's happening in our food industry. Supporting local farmers by going to the local market is not only trendy and social, it's one of the best things we can do for our health.

Educating people about how to manage the local food crops is just as important. I remember a friend on Whidbey Island, Washington, telling me that the local food kitchen was throwing away beautiful, fresh, organic vegetables because folks didn't know what they were or how to prepare them. That is how removed from nature many people are. In truth we aren't removed, we just don't know how connected we actually are, and how our lack of knowledge and clarity is wreaking havoc on our microbiomes.

In his bestseller *I Contain Multitudes: The Microbes Within Us and a Grander View of Life,* science writer Ed Yong quoted bacteriologist

Theodor Rosebury, who wrote about lab animals, "The germ-free animal is, by and large, a miserable creature, seeming at nearly every point to require an artificial substitute for the germs he lacks."[14] What if this statement applies also to those of us with dysbiotic modern Western microbiomes? What if the root cause of human disease isn't so much about genetic predisposition as it is failed symbiosis? What if a lack of colonies is at the root of an imbalance, or translocation of even symbiotic species to areas they shouldn't be, due to faulty lymphatic, immune, san jiao, mesentery, and digestive function? The microbiome plays a huge role in the pathology and physiology of Eastern medicine. Perhaps the primary reason it's been so difficult to conduct double-blind, placebo-controlled scientific studies of its concepts and remedies is that the microbiota, whose widespread existence, expression, and importance we are just beginning to recognize, plays such a major role in our individuality and health.

In their book, *The Hidden Half of Nature,* David Montgomery and Anne Bikle write that Linnaeus, considered the father of taxonomy, categorized microbes into the group infusoria, and put bacteria in the genus *Chaos.*[15] In a way, this is how our perception of the microbiome is at the moment: chaos. This is because we don't have a complete handle on every element in play, everything those critters manage, or how to control them. The strange irony is that we are conducting studies on sick people based upon the premise that the control is the perceived healthy microbiome of the contemporary Western European or North American human, which, as stated before, is much less diverse than that of our ancestors or modern-day people who live in, and according to, the cycles of nature.

This is why I propose we utilize the wisdom of Eastern medicine when learning exactly what we should be eating, how, why, when, and where, in order to support our microbiomes. This knowledge was developed at a time when people were living in nature, according to the cycles of nature. They had problems that required a medicine, but they also lived in harsh environments in the elements without modern conveniences like running water or antibiotics. Nonetheless there were centenarians, there were spiritually minded people, and there were athletes. But there probably weren't very many peanut allergies.

It is possible that the way our food is genetically modified and processed is confusing the intelligence of the body. This is what Eastern medicine recognizes. Processed or modified food is probably the number one problem when it comes to the confusion of the immune system regarding self and other, and what proteins are cause for concern and annihilation. The microbiome is intimately linked to this confusion, as it trains the immune system to recognize potential threats and act upon them. Eastern medicine may not be the panacea, as nothing is, but it does offer great insight lacking in modern medicine. Just ask anyone with symptoms that have stumped Western doctors who has achieved relief through Eastern medicine.

Functional medicine has similar ideas to many Eastern medicine concepts, such as being more aligned with nature, detoxifying the body, and so on. But it operates through the framework of Western medicine, and most functional medicine practitioners are either medical or osteopathic doctors who aren't trained in Eastern medicine. Even functional or naturopathic doctors use highly concentrated, pharmaceutical grade substances as opposed to simpler, bioavailable, more easily assimilable and less harsh substances in their whole form. And they don't have the contraindication knowledge of herb-herb interactions that Eastern medicine practitioners do. The Western and Eastern herbs standardized for Western consumers aren't all lab tested against one another, but Eastern medicine source texts include lists of contraindications for herbs used for certain presentations, or in formulas in tandem with one another.

Instead of trying to address a symptom or a disease, Eastern medicine is designed to support the body, partly through the balancing of the microbiome. It looks to the root of an imbalanced state and nudges the system into balance so a disease pattern can no longer thrive. It has an unwavering foundation and a universal lens through which it perceives reality, and this lens can be used to view, diagnose, and treat any individual. We don't treat diseases. Yes, diseases exist in Eastern medicine, but the ways they present are as unique as the individual. As Montgomery and Biklé put it, "culture shapes the questions people ask and how they interpret what they see."[16]

In Western culture there is the tendency to rely upon and shift from fad diet to fad diet. We don't need to go through each and every one of them here, although I would love it if someone did, but I think people need to understand how important it is to go back to basics and keep it simple instead of trying to constantly reinvent the wheel. When Eastern medicine practitioners are trained in diagnosis, we learn that if a pattern or series of patterns completely stumps us, what we should do is go back to basics. Instead of trying some fancy acupuncture treatment or medicinal therapy, isolate the simplest thing and start there. When things get so complex that we feel confused, what we need is to go back to the foundation we have in our root knowledge. This conveys simplicity to the client, whose body must be exhibiting confusion to the nth degree if we don't even know where to start with them. The body can then respond to the simplicity of treatment, and start to recalibrate itself from there. The same applies to diet and our digestion: We need to get back to basics. Nothing is bad; you are not one way all the time. Some things resonate, some things don't, and that changes at different times. Simplify in order to listen to yourself and understand what resonates and what doesn't. Favor what does, and if the body's strength or intelligence is weakened or confused, or you are unable to discern its messages, seek out someone who can help strengthen or clarify it and help you to reconnect.

What many are doing on a daily basis just isn't working. It is the rare exception when a person isn't burning the candle at both ends. Most of us don't feel we have time to cook regular meals, shop for fresh produce, spend time with our families or by ourselves, or even sleep, or maybe we just don't prioritize these things. The inexpensive, widely available foods we have easy access to are genetically modified, refrigerated, frozen, canned, precut, boxed, processed, and loaded with sugar and preservatives. If we want to change our microbiomes for the better, we need to reevaluate how we live. If we want to optimize and diversify our microbiomes, we need to make changes in our lives.

Self-care takeaways from this chapter:
- Include the five primary tastes in as many meals as possible.
- Avoid processed foods.
- Avoid refined sugar and flour.
- Switch to mineral rich salts (Himalayan pink or black salt).
- Add more dietary fiber.
- Eat whole-food oils that aren't processed.
- Steer away from fad diets.

7

Change Your Life, Change Your Microbiome
Restoring the Natural Intelligence of the Body

> *Before you heal someone, ask him if he's willing to give up the things that make him sick.*
>
> HIPPOCRATES

Given the yin and the yang in activity of our microbial counterparts and their metabolites, the key to a healthy self may not lie only or at all in supplementation. It may be that what we need to do is to restore the natural intelligence in the function of our human cells and in our microbes, the communication between the two, and the way the body benefits from them and their metabolites. This is a key concept in Eastern medicine. Prevention and treatment involve recognizing potential obstacles to the intelligent balance of the body and removing those factors. Obvious examples are to eliminate triggers, for example, gluten for someone with celiac disease or peanuts for someone with a peanut allergy.

These are extreme examples because the response to these triggers happens immediately in most cases. For other situations, the trigger may be something that is just pushing the person over the top of the homeostatic threshold. This could be an irritant, overindulgence in caffeine, alcohol, or anything for that matter, or how the person is eating. If eating is irregular or happens while the person is upset, these are also triggers. Other eating habits that may irritate digestion include eating before bed, overexposure to social media and close-up screens, the news, "toxic" behavior from others, or toxic thinking.

After the obstacle or primary trigger is removed, the system may need to be reset. How we do this is the trick. For some, the damage may be so deep that it may not be possible to fully reverse the disorder. This could be for a number of reasons, for example, a genetic predisposition that gets activated or the presence of unknown obstacles in the cascade of imbalance. Healing may be inhibited by inability to change a toxic job or work differently, or to eat well, or by the inability to afford optimal treatment, supplements, or medication. In a conversation with Buddhist spiritual teacher Lama Lhanang Rinpoche, we concluded the primary contributing factor is the mind. A stuck mental/emotional pattern, or an attachment to something that blocks the healing process deep within the psyche is probably the most difficult obstacle of all to overcome. It involves consistent attention and not only the resolve, but the willingness to be vulnerable and surrender to life and truth in order for a stuck mental pattern to be overcome. These we call not just karma, but *samskaras,* or patterns, in Eastern philosophy. They are tightly wound knots deep within the psyche and body.

The process of healing the gut, including the microbiome, may not only alleviate systemic or seemingly unrelated symptoms, but allow greater tolerance to triggers that previously would have brought on serious illness. I know several people who have been diagnosed with celiac disease who can now expose themselves to gut-barrier offenders like caffeine and alcohol, or can now tolerate minimal exposure to gluten on an irregular basis. It's interesting to note that I've had two clients who were diagnosed clinically with celiac disease but are able to eat gluten-containing products in Italy. This suggests to me that there may be more at play in American wheat than just gluten. Perhaps the genetic modifications have altered the surface of the protein, or maybe the body is reacting to pesticide residue, or some kind of fungal or microbial contamination during transport and storage. There may be a natural sensitivity, but perhaps it's the added assault that pushes the immune system over the edge.

Getting back to the current discussion, Eastern medicine doesn't stop at supplementation, and in Eastern medicine we generally don't leave people on supplements of any kind—teas, decoctions, pills, tinctures, powders, and so on—for more than a few months at a time. At least I usually don't. Supplements are always being tweaked because there are stages to the process of healing, and they vary from person to person. Either the initial trigger is removed, or the lacking substance added, and the body figures out how to right the situation on its own—or it needs to be given the space, or nudge, and resources to move to the next stage.

When the body is given the space and resources to heal, unless it's in a final stage of disease progression, it will usually do so. Having a good practitioner to assess what is still out of balance along the way is key. There are many variables to the process and they often combine into a confusing knot of information and activity that needs to be rooted out and carefully untangled. This is where the eight principles of diagnosis of Chinese medicine can be very useful (see the box on the facing page). Is the client's inner environment cold or hot, and where? Is it more yin or yang? Is the imbalance generated internally or is it the result of an external invader? As part of this line of questioning we ask to what degree and depth is the offender, and what is the best way to deal with it? And last, is the environment one of excess or deficiency? Maybe it's both. Perhaps there is excess manifesting in one place or way and deficiency in another. Assessment can be tricky and overwhelming and that is cause to seek out a highly regarded practitioner. This applies also to practitioners. We often try to treat ourselves, but it can be difficult to objectively self-assess.

So what do the Eastern medicine principles that directly influence the health of the microbiome actually entail in practice? The first, from

---

The Eight Principles of Chinese Medicine
Patterns of Disharmony

Eastern medicine relies not only on symptoms but also on patterns of disharmony in the body. These measure an excess or deficiency in the qi (vitality), blood, yin (fluids and substance), and yang (energetics, metabolism, and heat).

1. **Yin** is, generally speaking, cold, moist, stationary, and heavy.

2. **Yang** is warm, hot, rises up, and is mobile.

3. **Interior** refers to patterns that are generated from deep within the body and mind.

4. **Exterior** patterns are those that enter from outside of the body, such as an external pathogen.

5. **Heat** means there are excess heat signs and symptoms, such as a sensation of heat; red face, eyes, or skin; or inflammation.

6. **Cold** indicates a subjective aversion to cold, as well as other symptoms that may occur when cold is present, such as pain, oftentimes due to deficiency.

7. **Deficiency** describes inadequacy in the qi, blood, fluids, yin, yang, or essence.

8. **Excess** is used to describe a pattern where a bodily substance builds up. This can be an accumulation of qi, blood, fluids, yin, or yang. It can also point to one of the six excesses: wind, coldness, heat, dryness, dampness, or summerheat.

---

a diet perspective, is the recognition that all food is medicine and is not inherently bad, and, conversely, that all food can cause imbalance. The second is that each of us has innate tendencies that predispose us to having certain sensitivities. These sensitivities are not allergies or even clinical sensitivities, but subclinical sensitivities. These subclinical sensitivities are usually to foods we do best eating in moderation in order to keep our constitutional tendencies in balance. We receive subtle cues from our inner physician through our unique language of feelings, senses, intuitions, and outright messages. Messages often come through the quality of bowel movements, as we learned from chapter 3.

There is so much rich practical advice for improving health and potentially balancing the microbiome. There are studies on a smattering of these recommendations, and some have already been highlighted in the text. Others that aren't here are readily accessible via your nearest search engine. For example, do you want to know how coffee affects the microbiome? Input "coffee" and "microbiome." It turns out it's high in antioxidants and is actually a prebiotic said to help balance the liver; studies show that regular consumption may help reduce the risk of liver cancer and other liver diseases. I think we can assume that taken in moderation in small amounts, good quality coffee can have beneficial physiological effects. Remember, no food is inherently bad. In Chinese medicine, we say coffee "smooths the liver qi" in small quantities, less than six ounces a day. The same is true for wine and beer, which are also considered prebiotics, or food for our microbes, with positive healthful effects in moderation. In Eastern medicine we use wine to administer herbs under certain conditions, and on its own it is known to be warming and increase circulation, again in moderation. That means small, inconsistent doses.

I'm not advising loading up on alcohol and coffee. I am merely illustrating that according to both systems of medicine, Western and Eastern, there are recognized health benefits to even the highest offenders on the "do not consume" list of most diets. In addition, we are seeing that food can be used for good, or it can contribute to greater imbalance. Coffee in excess can aggravate the liver qi and cause nervousness and palpitations. Alcohol in excess creates an unsettled and confused mental state, and can have a multitude of negative consequences. Both can be detrimental in any amount to someone with a sensitivity, subclinical or otherwise, and in the cases of permeable gut walls, can increase that permeability.

There are innumerable studies that have yet to be done, or perhaps never will be done, on the influence on the microbiome of more specific aspects of lifestyle, mental activity, environment, and diet. For those activities we can combine the rudimentary knowledge we have about the microbiome, much of which is in the beginning of this book, with Eastern medicine principles about how the mind and body work and their relationship to the environment, and add personal experience and common sense to figure out how to balance it. Now that you have a grounding in the importance of the microbiome on your health, and are armed with the knowledge that there is a wisdom within you that is capable of great discernment and guidance, you can move forward with understanding the guidelines and practices that have been systematically outlined by the Eastern traditions over millennia.

The Lung-Large Intestine-Skin Axis

First, take a deep breath. Breathing well and staying aware of the breath helps us to detoxify about 70 percent of bodily toxins. Breathing well:

- Stimulates the vagus nerve
- Detoxifies the body
- Calms the mind
- Assists with lymphatic and other circulation
- Oxygenates the blood
- Brings clarity to the mind
- Stimulates the internal organs via diaphragmatic movement
- Harmonizes the san jiao
- Wrings out and moves the internal organs, including the mo yuan
- Massages the internal organs
- Enhances good posture
- Relieves secondary breathing muscle fatigue
- Energizes the body and mind
- Makes you feel good

In the chapter 1 discussion of the lung microbiome, we learned that although many of the inhabitants of that area are transient, there is consistency as to which microbes tend to be there. It is when there is an invader that the immune system is alerted and the inflammatory process starts. An infection is an alert that there is an overabundance of a pathogen or even too much of a beneficial microbe somewhere it shouldn't be. Keeping the lungs moving fully may help us to expel potential invaders, keep microbes from sticking, and keep the transients on the move. For all the reasons mentioned above, deep breathing is necessary for optimal immunity and to expel potential problems from the body. Deep diaphragmatic breathing also helps to clear heat from the lower body. When we breathe well we not only expel toxins that otherwise may stay in circulation, we also utilize efficient detoxification of the body without taxing the gut or the liver unnecessarily with the task.

The highest concentration of blood vessels to the lungs are in the lower lobes. If we aren't making optimal use of this area by doing deep, diaphragmatic breathing, we may not be completely oxygenating the blood or eliminating toxins. Chronic shallow or fast breathing into the chest using the neck, pecs, and upper-back muscles requires energy the body could be using for cleanup and rejuvenation. Instead we exhaust ourselves by being tense and not fully allowing air in or completely emptying our lungs on the out breath.

The liver is actually attached to the diaphragm. In Eastern medicine a major protocol for resolving imbalances is to keep the liver energies cool, calm, and easygoing. When it is stuck in position, not being squeezed and expanded by the diaphragm, vitality stagnates. We become cranky and frustrated, and digestion is oftentimes adversely affected. By breathing deeply, we enhance the mobility of all the internal structures, allowing for more complete circulation, detoxification, and transformation. Just like the body in general, organs and tissues that are soft, moist, warm (not hot), and toned are much healthier than those that are rigid, inflexible, inflamed, and lack tone. Well-respected Chinese

---

The Breath at Rest

It's important to add a note here about what a healthy, natural breath is. On average, it is optimal to be breathing 12–16 times per minute. Twelve times or below—especially in those practicing yoga or qigong, and barring some abnormality—is optimal. Anything above sixteen is considered a form of hyperventilation, or an indication that the nervous system is on high alert. I'd also like to make a distinction about shallow breathing. When at rest, it's normal to feel as if the breath is shallow. If the body doesn't require big breathing for physiological or activity related purposes, we should actually be taking effortless breaths that feel like they mainly enter the chest. The distinction I'd like to make is that there's a difference between this breathing, that may feel shallow because it isn't huge like a sigh or intentional belly breath, and fast breathing. I think a lot of the time we call what the breath is at rest shallow breathing, yet what we think of as the negative connotation of shallow breathing is actually accelerated breathing. This fast or quick breathing is the kind that utilizes accessory breathing muscles as opposed to the diaphragm as the primary breathing muscle.

---

medicine oncology expert and teacher Tai Lahans calls the diaphragm, "the dynamic heat exchanger" between the upper and lower jiao. This means that in Eastern medicine, inflammation can be alleviated or avoided to some extent by chronic, healthy movement of the diaphragm.

Holding in the belly is a common cause of chronic, shallow, fast breathing. We are indoctrinated to believe we need to have a flat abdomen to be attractive. At a young age, girls and boys alike start sucking in their bellies. This chronic holding may actually be sending a message to the brain that we aren't safe. Contracting the abdomen is an aspect of the fight-or-flight response, as it is a survival mechanism to protect the internal organs from trauma. It becomes problematic when we experience chronic stress because the constant low-grade fight-or-flight reactivity causes the belly to remain in a state of contraction. When this happens we unconsciously breathe more shallowly, quickly, and less efficiently and healthfully, and this chronic holding may have an adverse effect on gut function and the microbiome. The body, mind, and microbiome are affected by everything we do or don't do. Without a nice soft belly, particularly above the navel, that allows for the correct rhythmic movement of the diaphragm and orbit of excursion for the internal organs, it makes sense that all three will suffer.

There is an intimate connection between the lung and large intestine pathways in Eastern medicine. Speaking in terms of the shen (spirit), or consciousness, the lungs are responsible for the management of grief. Any grief can impede the optimal functioning of the lungs. The large intestine is tasked with being present and releasing, both metaphorically and literally. Grief is a holding; release is a letting go, the act of no longer grasping. One can see how these two are connected, grief and letting go, they are like two sides of the same coin. They both involve not dwelling in the past, but being in present-moment awareness. Even if there is grief, being present with it allows it to be processed. In that presence there is acceptance, and when there is acceptance there is a release.

When one organ isn't working well, another suffers. The lungs are tasked with sending vitality downward to help expel waste from the large intestine. If this isn't happening, oftentimes because of a held-in or tight abdomen and a rigid diaphragm with shallow or quick breathing, the elimination will suffer. This can lead to various forms of constipation. If the constipation is severe, heat may be created and rise up, unable to dissipate via diaphragmatic movement, and allow for greater stagnation of waste in the large intestine. If the large intestine cannot send vitality downward, it can restrict the downward movement of the vitality of the lungs as well. It's easy to see the vicious cycle that can occur with this dynamic and make way for an adverse change in microbial balance in the large intestine. If there is stagnation in the large intestine the lungs can't do their job well, and this may result in subpar lung function, as mentioned above.

Thanks to studies done thus far on the human exposome, we know that exhaled microbial metabolites can be measured and linked to the metabolites produced by the microbial inhabitants colonizing the large intestine.[1] In addition to a link between the lungs and large intestine in Eastern medicine, there is a strong link between them both and the skin. Toxins that build in the large intestine will often manifest as skin issues. If the energetics of the lungs are not optimal, the energetic or spirit that animates them fully, called the *po,* can float outward toward the skin and make the skin, via the nervous system, more sensitive. If the large intestine is adversely affected by too much mental activity, this nervous-system disruption may manifest as a vata imbalance, or imbalance of air in the system. This can be experienced as flightiness, dryness, nervousness, jitters, inability to sit still, constant movement, insomnia, or anxiety. The skin can also be diagnostic for the state of the physical form of the large intestine. According to a translation of the Ling Shu, or *Spiritual Axis,* by late Chinese medicine expert Giovanni Maciocia, the condition of the skin reflects the inner landscape of the large intestine. For example, when the skin is tight, it can mean that the large intestine is tight, too, also the thickness of the skin reflects the thickness or thinness of the large intestine walls.[2]

If we want to clean ourselves, we bathe. To clean our insides we drink pure water, breathe clean air, and eat whole foods. Likewise we should nourish our skin, apply rubbing techniques and pure oils, and avoid products with added chemical surfactants and other possible irritants. This is important to the skin microbiome and metabolome. The metabolome of the skin includes all the by-products or metabolites of the cells and microbes that serve as chemical messengers and regulators of bodily functions, such as hormones and the like.[3] It also includes the molecules left as residue on the skin that may interfere with cell-to-cell and microbe-to-cell messaging, such as additives in skin lotion, shampoo, hair treatments, cosmetics, and perfume.[4] We should actually be feeding the skin microbiome with what we apply, not disturbing its balance.

To cleanse and balance our lungs and large intestine, including the microbiome, and nourish them and it, we need to breathe well, inhaling fresh, clean air (as opposed to stagnant air) as often as possible. The lungs are partially nourished by the diversity of microbes we breathe, as the gut microbiome, largely in the large intestine, is nourished by the diversity of foods we eat.

The Breath Is the Bridge

The breath is the bridge between the body and our conscious awareness, between the body and our vitality, between the body and the mind, and between the body and our awareness of truth. The breath also connects us to the consciousness and memories anchored in the bodily tissues. The first step to breathing well for you and your microbiome is to be a good listener and accept what it is that your body is saying.

Yogavisharada B.N.S. Iyengar teaches that the lungs are like a rich web. This web needs to be gently stretched over time or it will be damaged by making it do more than it has the resiliency for in the moment. Iyengar was talking about breath control techniques, or pranayama practices, but it is the same with even the most seemingly innocuous deep breath that we demand of ourselves, believing we "should" be able to do it even if we can't. If a deep breath feels constricted and inhaling is causing stress, forcing it is not making progress toward optimal healthy breathing. Instead, it may be creating an obstacle to that end.

It may sound too simple to acknowledge the power of the breath, especially when there is no evidence of lung disease, so the assumption is that the breath is just fine. I think most people will find that it is not. Either they are uncomfortable with focusing on it or will find there is an imbalance on a gross or subtle level. There is an inherent vulnerability in opening to and accepting the breath as it is in the moment. Many messages from the body and mind are often hidden beneath the breath, beneath the diaphragm. Focusing on the breath allows these messages to percolate to the surface of the awareness, and although the breath brings a sense of spaciousness, the messages can be accompanied by a myriad of uncomfortable memories, feelings, and bodily sensations. This is part of healing, allowing for the polarity inherent in life, the grasping and the release, to manifest in whatever way is needed.

In chapter 5 we touched upon the five spirits, or mental/emotional aspects of consciousness seated in the body. The body is the anchor and the vehicle for the experience of these states of awareness and emotion. The breath integrates the body with the less tangible parts of our existence: our bodily consciousness, our vitality, our mind and emotions, and our truth. This is why yogis practice breath awareness and control exercises. They are simultaneously increasing awareness, spaciousness, and connection to intuition or inner knowing while intentionally directing their vitality. Martial artists do this as well. Whether internal (managing one's own vitality) or external (involving interaction with another's vitality) martial arts, there is some aspect of breath awareness and using the breath to direct qi or vitality. Actor and martial artist Bruce Lee was an exceptional example of this. He moved with grace and fluidity, speed and great agility. He was able to perceive what his opponent would do a split second before the person even initiated the movement. Science has acknowledged that we are actually perceiving reality a split second after it manifests. Ask any acupuncturist how this works. Often before the client reacts to feeling the connection to, movement, or rush of qi while being needled, the practitioner can feel it. This is true present-moment awareness. These traits were not intrinsic to Bruce Lee, nor did he acquire them solely by brute bodily practices. He internally focused on the wisdom and mystery of being—on the breath—and recognized the importance of self-knowledge and the connection to all that is.

The conscious awareness or experience of this connection can be realized through the intention of breath awareness practice and paying attention to feelings and emotions. They can teach us, and always do if we listen and allow.

⇒·⇐

Breath Awareness Practice

There are many things at play with the breath. You must utilize your presence and objective awareness, as well as your ability to release expectations and attachment to things being a certain way, and make space for the wise teacher within you, your inner physician, to come through and gently coax the breath into a healthier pattern.

- Please read through this section entirely before practice. Set aside several minutes a day to observe your breathing. Get comfortable. Take five deep breaths and notice how you feel. If it is uncomfortable, abandon trying to take deep breaths at all right now. Simply breathe in a way that feels comfortable and allow for the space within yourself to open. You may need to work up to deeper breaths over time, and that is perfectly fine. You can continue with the rest of the practice from where your breath currently is. If a part of it feels too challenging or causes anxiety, back off and go back to simply observing the following.
- Sit, breathe, feel, and allow. Let yourself feel your breath as it is in the moment. Feel where it enters and where it goes. Feel the boundary around it inside your body. Is it in the chest? Where? Do your ribs feel encased in a vise grip? Does the air float effortlessly in and out or is there some conscious involvement from you? Are you judging it or merely observing it? Move from judge to observer. Observe sensation. Allow only what is.
- As you observe the breath, note that it may begin to slow some, and that the boundary around where it lands in the body begins to gently stretch, expand, or become more diffuse. You may stay in this phase of the practice for days or even weeks.
- The breathing pattern involves the inhale, the transition between the inhalation and exhalation, an exhale, and a pause. Focus on this pattern for a few minutes. Notice anything you can about what each phase of the breathing cycle feels like to you. What feels most comfortable, what least comfortable?

❦ Now that you've done this for a few minutes, bring your awareness back to how the breath feels coming in through your nose and where it goes in the body. How does your body feel around these areas? Does it feel easier now? More spacious? Play with the edges of the space. See if the border around it can start to expand, dissolve, or spread out. Play with this for a few minutes.

❦ Now let's get the mind involved more actively. Ideally the breath comes in through the nose and moves like a wave through the torso. If you are lying down, put your hands on your abdomen, one on the navel, one on the chest. Feel the breath wave as it moves through you. What does it feel like? Do you feel the bottom hand lift first on the inhale and then the top hand, or is it the other way around? Does the bottom hand lower first on the exhale, or the top one? In an unobstructed, rhythmically appropriate, healthy breath pattern, the bottom hand should lift first on the inhale and drop first on the exhale. This means that the diaphragm is moving properly as the instigator of the breathing, as opposed to the secondary breathing muscles. If the diaphragm is moving properly, the body follows. This means the ribcage slightly opens and lifts at the bottom to allow room for the diaphragm to travel downward like an inverted umbrella, and closes around it like a hug as it travels back up on the exhale. If the opposite happens, you are reverse breathing.

Reverse breathing is a technique in internal martial arts and advanced yoga practices that is done temporarily and intentionally to achieve a specific response. When it is done unconsciously by people who aren't advanced practitioners being guided by a qualified teacher, it may create a disturbance in the mind. I was unable to locate any specific research on the gut microbiome–brain connection in relationship to breathing, other than that studied on specific microbial populations in the lungs in diseased vs. healthy states. It makes sense, though, that since every single thing we do affects the microbiome somehow, and since there is communication via the vagus nerve between the brain and the gut microbiome, that the timing and rhythm of the diaphragm during the breathing cycle would have an impact on what messages are being communicated and how the body's reactions to them are making us feel.

It is not uncommon for a reverse breathing pattern, or fast, shallow breathing pattern, to be accompanied by such ailments as generalized anxiety, jaw clenching, teeth grinding, panic attacks, insomnia, and a sense of overwhelm or reduced stress tolerance. No doubt the microbiome plays a role in this. Anyone with experience in breathing patterns and having a well-developed sense of embodiment with the breath will acknowledge that the breath is just as important as what you're putting in your mouth.

Once you've spent a few weeks observing and practicing the allowing with only the slight interference of expanding the breath boundaries, you can begin working on the wave pattern. Like the spaciousness that happens in the body when the breath comes in, the wave is not well defined. I am dividing it here into parts, but really, it should end up feeling like the body is moving all at once with the breath, like there is no dividing line. We focus on a two-part wave action here for simplicity's sake, but you may find that it is more like three-part wave action, and far more involved than that, that it feels like it is all moving at once, and that it involves the entire length of the spine and the structures attached to it.

> ❧ After doing the spaciousness practice for a few weeks, transition to the wave phase more intently. Bring awareness to both hands to start. Feel them rise on the inhale, and drop on the exhale. Lift when you breathe in, lower when you breathe out. Do this for 10 to 20 breaths.
> ❧ Now note how your wave is moving. Do this for another 10 breaths.
> ❧ Let it shift slowly, over the course of another 10 to 20 breaths, to one where the bottom hand lifts on the inhale, then the top hand. On the exhale, let the bottom hand lower first, then the top hand. Once this pattern is comfortably established, let go of trying to do anything and just go back to a relaxed breathing pattern, where you feel peaceful and don't care what your breathing is doing.

Over time this practice will bring whatever needs to be redirected or cleared from your circuitry and bodily tissues to the surface awareness for processing. All the while everything will be shifting toward a more healthful state of being in body, mind, spirit, and microbiome.

By slowly reorganizing the breathing pattern and increasing awareness, unlimited sensations, memories, and internal experiences will manifest. In the process, unexpected things may begin to change: better sleep, outer glow, improved digestion, shifting perspective, greater sense of well-being and tolerance of stress, less anxiety, and more spontaneous presence, appreciation, and joy.

The Science of Cycles

Being aware of cycles of time such as life span, solar cycle, year with its seasonal influences and observances, lunar cycle/month, and daily cycle are foundational in Eastern medicine theory, so I devoted a whole chapter to this topic in my previous book. There is a current in nature that ebbs and flows, and its waves lap upon the surface of the other cycles. All of the cycles are occurring simultaneously, like latitude, longitude, and time intersecting at the core of each living being. For our purposes here, we will talk about the seasonal cycles and daily cycles, and how the microbiome changes within these.

Just as birds and butterflies have an internal timing device that tells them when to migrate for the season, so do humans. It's called a biological clock and is part of an entire field of biological processes.[5] There are several cycles recognized within this field:

- Circadian rhythms, sleep/wake cycles, occur once every 24 hours. Body temperature is a part of this cycle.
- Infradian rhythms repeat over periods longer than 24 hours, for example, hibernation in bears, or the menstrual cycle.
- Ultradian cycles are those that occur repeatedly in a 24-hour day. They include the respiratory rhythm, the different aspects of the sleep cycle, and when is best to eat food.[6] And for the yogis

reading this, the ultradian rhythm seems to align with *swara,* or the yogic science of rest and activity, and which *nadi,* or channel of vitality, is dominant in any period of time throughout the day.

In Ayurveda the infradian rhythm is recognized in what's called *ritucharya,* or yearly/seasonal cycles. In Eastern medicine we recognize eating according to the season as an aspect of ritucharya.

Daily cycles, which include the circadian rhythm and the ultradian rhythm, are called *dinacharya,* or daily routine. Eating at specific windows of time during the day is an aspect of dinacharya. You don't need to remember the Sanskrit terminology, as the guidelines are present regardless of which Eastern medical tradition you consult. The point is that knowledge of these cycles existed long before now, along with an awareness of the resulting imbalances that occur from not attending to them.

With regard to seasonal cycles, it is recommended to eat according to what is naturally available at any given time of year. Of course, those of us fortunate to have plentiful access to pretty much everything all year long will also choose foods that are not in season. Nonetheless, the body knows what is best for it at particular times. Dr. John Douillard explains this beautifully in articles on his LifeSpa website, as well as in his books. According to Douillard, the gut microbiome changes in time with the shift in seasons, readying us to digest the foods that are widely available.[7] He describes three seasons of growing and harvesting and one season of dormancy, and outlines which foods are most appropriate in which seasons.

Winter: Nuts, seeds, meats, and more fat and protein are advisable.

Spring: Eat a low-fat diet full of leafy greens and berries.

Summer: Gravitate toward cooling, high-carbohydrate fruits and veggies.[8]

Autumn: I recommend seasonal harvest foods with lots of easy-to-digest, nourishing broths and stews.

Living beings—including our microorganisms—have biological clocks and rhythms. A study done on blue-green algae confirmed this. In humans, the 24-hour circadian rhythm, specifically the sleep/wake cycle, is believed to be regulated by exposure to darkness and light, and the activity of melatonin. In algae, though, it was found that although light exposure can reset their rhythm if it is thrown off, they largely regulate themselves according to metabolic signaling, through the circulation of ATP (adenosine triphosphate, the energy-carrying molecule) and ADP (adenosine diphosphate, also an energy-carrying molecule).[9] Humans, on the other hand, have a built in sleep-wake cycle based upon sunlight. Recently this knowledge was confirmed by Nobel

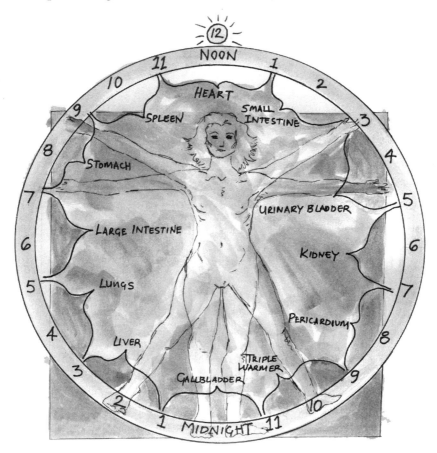

This image illustrates the circadian clock.

Prize–winning circadian clock researchers who described the molecular cause of the internal clock. They found a gene that makes a protein that builds up inside cells during the day, but degrades at night.[10] These day/night rhythms affect everything from how the body metabolizes food to behavior, hormonal activity, body temperature, and sleep.[11] See diagram (p. 165) for how the daily clock influences the mind and body.

The Night/Day Cycle

Many of us have heard of melatonin, and that it is related to sleep. It is a hormone that the brain secretes in response to lack of sunlight, and it changes with the seasons.[12] This is aligned with Eastern medicine and the solar cycle, which brings changes in our physiology throughout the year. In terms of sleep, melatonin secretion begins when the sun goes down. Its duration lengthens in winter and gets shorter in summer in response to the presence of more sunlight.[13] Its secretion begins around 9:00 p.m. and subsides as daylight hours begin, by 7:30 in the morning.[14]

Eastern medicine teaches that we should be asleep just after dark, and definitely by 10:00 p.m., and that we should wake up before melatonin secretion subsides completely, or between 5:00 and 7:00 a.m. Going to bed after 10:00 p.m. can cause a second wind and difficulty falling asleep. Waking up later in the morning or sleeping well beyond the cessation of melatonin secretion can cause one to feel groggy and foggy. Blue light from technical devices is renowned for interfering with the sleep/wake cycle. Good sleep hygiene, therefore, involves not only going to bed before 10:00, but limiting exposure to blue light in the preceding time period. Most devices now have blue-light dimmers built into the settings. If you must be up late on a backlit device, it is best to use this setting. Opticians often recommend blue-light inhibitors in prescription lenses. However, if blue light is partially responsible for inhibiting melatonin production, then wearing these all day may send the body the wrong signal. It may be more beneficial to have two pairs of glasses, a pair to be worn during the day when you want blue light to help keep you awake, and blue light–blocking glasses for the evening to allow the body to naturally adjust to the absence of light.

What does all of this have to do with the microbiome? Quite a bit, actually. I mentioned in the introduction that certain microbes are activated by metabolism, but by and large, metabolism is activated by the sleep/wake cycle, including the activity of the microbiome. The microbiome is influenced not only by what we eat but by when we eat.[15] To foster a greater diversity of microbes, eating is recommended during daylight hours only, more in the morning and less later in the day.[16] In the book *What to Eat When,* Dr. Michael Roizen and his coauthors, Michael Crupain and Ted Spiker, cite studies conducted on gut microbiomes and the influence of the circadian clock showing that gut flora are more active early in the day, and less so at night. During the early part of the day they influence the body to metabolize and grow cells. In the evening and at night they influence genes that put the body into detoxification mode.[17]

In addition, people who eat closer to 8:00 p.m. or later are more insulin resistant.[18] This indicates the body doesn't metabolize glucose the same way at night as it does during the day, and stores it as fat. Glucose is best metabolized during the early part of the day, when the body is most active and the muscles need energy.[19] This could mean that a preventive measure for prediabetes and a lifestyle adjustment for diabetics may be to change when, not just what, they are eating. The highest energy time of the day is between 10:00 a.m. and 5:00 p.m.[20] This means we should be consuming the majority of our food between these hours. In fact, Eastern teachings emphasize the importance of eating our largest meal either in the morning or for lunch. This is when the body has the most strength and ability to burn the most calories. The strength of our digestion is greatest when the sun is at its peak. As above, so below. Between midmorning and early afternoon is when the function of the spleen qi/agni/digestive fire is at its height for the day.

Eastern medicine has recognized this for centuries. For yogis and serious meditators, most of their food is "front-ended" to the early daylight hours. Lama Lhanang Rinpoche once told me that in monasteries the monks stop eating around noon. They are on a schedule that follows the daylight. It isn't just that they are living according to the light, however. They believe that we house millions of living entities in our bodies that are most active in the morning. The activity of these entities begins declining by noon, or very soon after that. Lama told me that eating later than that is not good for these sentient beings because they may become overwhelmed or overburdened by a heavy meal when their energy is waning. *Ahimsa,* or refraining from harming any living being, is both a yogic and Buddhist principle, and it includes our microbiome and ourselves. It is a form of subtle violence to violate the natural laws that, if followed, keep us and our precious little entities thriving.

This one anecdote may not be enough to cause most people to want to change when they eat, or even the awareness of the scientific backing of the practice of front-ending meals. What is undeniable is firsthand experience. When I was growing up, my family ate dinner between 5:00 and 6:00 p.m. every night, as did most of the other families in my neighborhood, so this is achievable. Try not eating at night for a few weeks, then try having your largest meal for breakfast or lunch. This may mean hot cereal like oatmeal for dinner, and a dinner meal for breakfast. Another option is to make your largest meal of the day lunch, and have something broth-based or easily digestible for dinner. You could also try having a small portion of food for dinner, maybe half what you'd normally eat. If you're waiting for someone to come home to eat who normally eats at 8:00 p.m. or later, just have tea while you sit together. Or if this is your usual dinner time, have something light, such as broth or thin, cooked cereal that's easy to digest. There are ways to eat in better alignment with your body and the natural cycles that require more mental determination than anything else. Give it a try for two weeks and see for yourself. Chances are that you'll discover the real obstacle to living more harmoniously arises from habits, outdated beliefs, and the stubbornness of one's own mind.

Before leading clients in a "cleanse," which I prefer to call a "dietary reset," I usually do one myself. The last time I did this I bumped up the time for dinner to happen between 4:00 and 5:30 p.m. at the latest, and had something very light. If I felt hungry later, I had some tea, and that usually took care of it, or I ate something healthy and small. Within two weeks I couldn't go through a day at work without people telling me how good I looked. I felt lighter and had more energy, slept better, had fewer cravings, and was satiated with simple foods. I also realized how much my mind and bad habits had to do with eating late, eating too much, and eating things I really shouldn't. I will outline a customizable dietary reset regimen in the next chapter.

Another circadian guideline recognized centuries ago in the East is to go to bed earlier. The old adage is that every hour of sleep one gets before midnight is like two hours compared to the hours after. This is true according to the organ clock. By the time 10:00 p.m. rolls around, if we aren't asleep, we are prone to a second wind. This is a time when we should be fast asleep, as our deepest sleep occurs by 2:00 a.m., and melatonin starts decreasing and shuts off by 7:30 a.m. According to the organ clock of Eastern medicines, detoxification mode amps up by 10:00 p.m. This means that if we aren't already asleep, not only do we not enter fully into scavenge and detox mode, we may actually start ingesting things again. We also may not get the optimal predeepest sleep hours in to allow for deep, restful, rejuvenating sleep. The hours from 1:00 to 3:00 a.m. are liver time. This is when the liver energy is dominant and the liver is hard at work cleaning our blood of toxins. If we aren't deeply asleep for this, we may be missing out on a massive boon to our health, and possibly setting ourselves up for imbalance. I can't count how many people are awake between these hours, either because they haven't fallen asleep yet or because they've woken up during this time and are often unable to get back to sleep. If the liver energy is taxed or is lacking in any fluids or nutrition, the vitality and consciousness of the liver cannot be peaceful. They rise up and wake us, letting us know that there is an imbalance here. We need to go to bed earlier, stop eating before dark (or ideally, dusk), avoid liver-aggravating food and drink, adopt a good bedtime ritual, or practice liver soothing and smoothing practices such as breath work, gentle yoga, or meditation, or some combination of all of the above. There is evidence that poor or disturbed sleep adversely affects the diversity of the microbiome.[21] Sadly enough, it takes only two days of disturbed or inadequate sleep in a row to start decreasing beneficial flora counts in the gut.[22]

> The main takeaways from this chapter for optimizing your health by nourishing you and your microbial inhabitants are to:
> - Breathe well.
> - Reduce stress.
> - Use natural skin products.
> - Eat nourishing foods.
> - Eat earlier.
> - Sleep better.
> - Sleep earlier.

8

Dietary Reset Protocol

Eastern Practices for Internal Balance

All we have to do is decide what to do with the time that is given to us.

J. R. R. TOLKIEN

I call the process of making health-based food and lifestyle changes a dietary reset because I don't want it to be associated with a fad diet, cleanse, or detox. This is a process that most people can undergo in order to get to know their bodies, minds, habits, and beliefs better. It is centered around observing one's own digestion and metabolism, food habits and cravings, and recognizing what works and what doesn't to keep one well. This is a doable take on centuries of guidelnes on how to heal the mind and body. One simply needs to modify daily routines and habits. It can be implemented safely, seasonally, yearly, or whenever one feels the need.

I've designed this dietary reset to adhere to the traditional wisdom of Eastern medicine and Ayurvedic home-cleansing protocols. It does not eliminate groups such as carbs, grains, or legumes the way many diets or cleanses often do. Instead, it incorporates them in a way that increases long-term overall well-being, and shows people firsthand that most of them can eat these foods, feel good, and maybe even lose weight.

I developed this reset based on the research I did for this book on the microbiome, and as an answer to what we can do to keep it diverse and, therefore, healthy. I have found many similarities between Eastern medicine teachings and scientific research on the microbiome pertaining to which foods to favor, which to avoid, and biological rhythms. That information is summarized here.

What It Entails

This reset is flexible. What you eat may be incredibly varied, or very streamlined. That is up to you. It is simple, and although recommended here for seven to ten days, may actually be done over a weekend, or whenever you're feeling like you need it. I recommend doing a reset with the change of seasons as the body is already shifting then and the dietary recommendations here require less from the body. The lifestyle recommendations provide stability. They also increase mind-body awareness, lymphatic circulation, and natural detoxification. The primary dishes for this reset are simple staple meals from the East: kitchari and congee. Kitchari is a blend of split yellow mung beans and either white basmati rice or sona masoori rice; congee is a rice porridge—further explanation and recipes are provided on pages 194–98. If you are drawn to a strict Ayurvedic-inspired reset protocol, just eat kitchari three times a day. If you want to mix it up, eat kitchari for one or two meals and congee for the other(s).

Some people may not like kitchari; others may be in a state of gut healing that requires a break from all legumes. If this is the case, congee is an excellent substitute. If eating congee for every meal, I recommend limiting the reset to no more than three days and easing up a great deal on activity levels. With the kitchari, there is a complete protein. With congee, there is not. Some other bean or animal product, such as bone broth or egg, can be added to the congee. If you are adding eggs or meat, the reset may be done longer.

Vegetables are an important part of this dietary reset. I recommend leaning toward seasonal, local, organic veggies. They may be steamed, lightly sautéed, cooked right into the dish, or roasted and eaten with each meal. Since it is advisable to build up to eating thirty different plant foods a week to feed your microbes, this is a great time to start. The rice and mung beans in the kitchari are two plants, now twenty-eight to go, building to thirty slowly over the next few weeks—not just during the reset—and then it becomes a habit. Start out by including spices and herbs in this tally. Although I don't recommend nuts and seeds during the reset, I do after it. I like to sprinkle sesame seeds on most savory dishes. Fruits are also not off the table for the reset, but should be eaten whole, and an hour before or two hours after any meal. This is because the fruit ferments quickly in the body and we don't want it sitting and rotting on top of the things that will be in the stomach for a longer time frame.

The primary focus of this reset is to gently begin to move the gut microbiome to a greater state of diversity, heal the gut lining, and strengthen the vitality. To do this, we need to get out of the way of the body's natural ability to heal itself. This involves regular routine, self-reflection, and foods that are easy to digest. From there, we can build our lives on these principles and continue on the path of cultivating the microbiome postcleanse with an even more varied diet; intuitive and seasonal food choices; qi cultivation practices, such as meditation, qigong, and yoga; continued self-reflection and emotional awareness, feeling more embodied and empowered.

The Body Detoxifies Itself

Toxins in Eastern medicine can be the result of environmental exposure, mental or emotional molecules and residue trapped in the body, ingested toxins, or the result of inadequate digestive capacity for the diet or the way one is eating. This means that the vitality of the spleen, either cellularly or in the digestive tract, is not optimal, or that the strength of the agni is not balanced on a micro or macro level, and residue builds up. It can be in the GI tract or in any other tissue of the

Self-Assessment

When thinking of a cleanse or detox, what images come to mind? What does a cleanse mean to you? What do you need to remove? What is the fundamental underlying belief that fuels the need to cleanse yourself? One of the most important things we can do before embarking on a life change is to ask ourselves where the impetus for it is coming from. Look at what the primary driving force is that compels you to want to do a diet, cleanse, or detox. Is there a sense something is off? Do you want to lose weight? Do you dislike how you look? How you feel? What is the actual problem? My recommendation is to contemplate these things and be honest, and try not to judge or defend your answers. Then come at the potential for a cleanse or a detox from the perspective that you want more clarity, greater quality of life, and longevity.

The next question that comes up is, "What should I do?" There are so many books and diet gurus standing on a soapbox or popping up on mainstream and social media. The amount and content of the information we have access to is overwhelming and often conflicting. This is where this Eastern medicine–based dietary reset comes in. It doesn't count on the latest this, that, or bestseller, but on information grounded in thousands of years of tradition and successful practice. Fad diets and cleanses are done at the risk of setting the body out of balance because they take only a small part of the picture into consideration. Most of these diets are either trying to limit calories or burn fat, or remove potential inflammatory food groups, real or imagined, that are often blamed for "leaky gut." Often the health seeker flounders alone and ends up resorting back to old patterns before getting on the next diet bandwagon. It's a never-ending cycle because the whole person isn't addressed. Dietary guidelines rooted in Eastern teachings take into consideration all facets of lifestyle, eating and food, seasons and circadian rhythms, and individual qualities.

body. Wherever the vitality is weakest, it will manifest. When this happens a slimy film can accrue and spread, also to other parts of the body. If the stools are sticky, heavy, and stick to the toilet, or if there is a thick or allover coating on your tongue, you have toxins in your system. In Eastern medicine they are called ama, dampness, phlegm, or damp heat. Damp heat is when the yucky residue mixes with or causes heat or inflammation. These residues or toxins can be deeply buried or more superficial; more solid and tangible, or invisible like a mist that clouds the sensory orifices and the mind. From a more Western perspective these residues may manifest as candida overgrowth, biofilm, elevated cholesterol levels, brain fog, mucus, plaque, or any other substance we not only don't want in our systems, but don't want in overabundance or building up where they don't belong. They are things that cause us to be too cold, hot, dry, wet, lacking in vitality, or living with chronic inflammation.

When someone does a cleanse, fast, or dietary reset, there are processes that unfold in both body and mind. The body can undergo a shock, or it can be gently eased into the transition. What we want to do is start prepping the body to do what it already does naturally when we get ourselves and our habits out of the way: detoxify itself. This is a very important concept to grasp. The body doesn't need you to detoxify it or cleanse it. It only needs you to let up on what it is you do that inhibits it from doing so! It does a fine job without prohibitive, intense fasts or cleanses, or thousands of dollars of supplements and juicers. If it didn't, you wouldn't be here. Period. It cleanses us of toxins and impurities just fine on its own through the microbiome, organs and associated tissues of the lungs and large intestine, liver and gallbladder, and kidneys and bladder. By removing obstacles to the optimal functioning of the digestive tube and its accessory organs, we can optimize our food intake and allow for better breakdown and assimilation of food and nutrients. This gives the body the energy it needs to put into cleanup and repair, so it can scrape away, draw out, transform, and expel the toxins. In addition, by tailoring the diet to beneficial microbe-friendly foods, we are potentially taking the load off overworked organs, increasing anti-inflammatory actions in the body, and changing how we feel emotionally for the better.

In Eastern medicine dietary reset protocols, we begin by eliminating offending substances and habits surrounding diet and lifestyle. This gives the body a chance to ease into greater cleansing slowly, without doing anything drastic. By first eliminating foods that may be crutches for us, that we rely upon to speed up digestion or the brain, or that artificially speed up intestinal transit, we can get a good handle on exactly what our transit time is and how what we are eating can affect it. This way we clear out variables and simplify so that the body can work better on its own with minimal interference. For this dietary reset I recommend people start letting go of caffeine, alcohol, processed foods, refined sugar, refined flour, meat, dairy, eggs, nuts and seeds, and hot spices a week or so before beginning the simple diet they will be on while they're resetting their systems in the next part of the process. These things don't need to be eliminated permanently, although a life without caffeine, alcohol, or refined products certainly wouldn't hurt anyone. I recommend these things be removed temporarily so that any potential impediments to clearly observing one's metabolic type or digestive capacity are minimized.

Meat can take four days to travel through the GI tract, so keep that in mind. It may be one of the first things to remove as you begin the process. Someone addicted to sugar or caffeine may need a couple of weeks to wean off them, and it won't be comfortable; caffeine withdrawal can bring on headaches and fatigue. After this, whatever emotions were being masked by the caffeine start to percolate. Usually people realize they've been feeling a little sad or depressed, or have some grief issues that have been stuck on the back burner behind the hustle and bustle of daily living. The sugar detox can make people feel tired and cranky, and for some, causes body aches for days like they're coming down with the flu. During the reset, energy levels normalize throughout the day and the dips that triggered sugar cravings are much less pronounced, if existent at all.

For most people reading this, alcohol, dairy, and refined flour can be more of an irregular habit or preference. Eliminating them most likely won't lead to a detox reaction, although it may become obvious they've been used to alleviate emotional discomfort. This is an aspect of the mental/emotional part of the dietary reset. In the same way the body starts to readjust to not having these things, so does the mind. The process of going through this period of self-awareness brings recognition of just how powerful the pull of the mind really is, and how much it has to do with creating obstacles to change.

Again, I recommend easing into the transition of this dietary discovery by taking a week or two to first start decreasing, then temporarily eliminating from the diet potential irritants or substances that may interfere with gut transit. This is because we want the body to get used to what it feels like, on its own, without these things, and then readjust. Also, these foods can have unrecognized consequences when built up in the system due to regular consumption or overconsumption, including heaviness, fogginess, lack of concentration, energy peaks and valleys, waking at night, feeling anxious, and any number of digestive complaints, from bloating and gas to reflux, abdominal cramping, loose bowel movements, constipation, or feeling like something just isn't right.

Many fasts, cleanses, detoxes, and so on encourage abstaining from food, or consuming things that speed up digestion. When you're pooping out everything you've eaten in record time, you feel lighter and "cleaned out." This may be a good sensation temporarily, but it isn't a permanent fix and it gives no clear indication of what's actually going on with the metabolism or digestion. Once regular eating is resumed, it is only a matter of time before things go back to how they were before the "cleanse." I feel we need to get away from thinking that pooping our brains out is a desired outcome of cleansing. It is not. (Maybe it's called pooping our brains out for a reason.) It is actually a therapeutic modality called "purgation" in Eastern medicine, and should be administered only in the presence of certain imbalances or conditions in people who really need it. If done unnecessarily or even contrary to a person's constitutional tendencies or bodily strength, it can make an imbalance even worse, or lead to other issues.

Trendy "diets" recommend avoiding certain food groups entirely, and often permanently. When we avoid whole foods entirely or permanently there may be a number of undesired consequences. One, obviously, is that you are stopping yourself and your beneficial microbes from having something you may actually enjoy, and they may need. Another is that by just removing something that may be more difficult for you to digest, you aren't getting to the bottom of what's actually happening internally, and may be missing an opportunity to address a greater aspect of healing and repair. Often people remove entire food groups needlessly. Sometimes it's a necessity, but I can say from my experience that this isn't the norm.

It may also be that it isn't necessary to eat certain food groups all the time. I mentioned already the seasonal shifts that occur in nature and in our guts, which call for certain macromolecules or food types to be eaten with greater abundance. There are also cultural dietary recommendations that reflect the awareness that the body is better served by having foods in moderation. One example of this is called *ekadashi,* which means "eleven." This is largely a Hindu tradition of abstaining from grains on two days of every month, the eleventh day after the new moon, and the eleventh day after the full moon. On those days heavier foods are avoided in order to increase inner listening and intuition. The avoided foods include grains and legumes. Since those observing ekadashi are already vegetarian, those of us who aren't would also eliminate meat.

Followed by adherents of certain lineages within Hinduism and Jainism, regular fasting or partial fasting may be a practice rooted in long-forgotten wisdom hidden in Indian mythology. Hindus practicing ekadashi focus on the Indian mythological deity Vishnu, who is the sustainer in the Indian trinity and protects the universe from being destroyed.

Stories, I am finding, are rarely, if ever, just stories. There is usually truth contained within them. Abstaining from grains on two specific days each month may add to digestive integrity. In *Clean Gut* Dr. Junger encourages omitting grains for two to four days a month in order to maintain gut integrity.[1] For many of us, eating grains in moderation may give a break from them that promotes health without depriving ourselves and our microbial inhabitants of the beneficial effects of their consumption. But having them every day may be problematic and a major contributing factor to those who feel foggy after eating. It isn't advisable to remove them entirely as grains are actually an excellent prebiotic or food for beneficial microbes in the gut. Those adhering to a low FODMAP diet or no-grain diet may be implementing a grain of truth (pun intended) into their daily routine: that it is advisable to release these things from the diet on a regular, although limited basis. However, the rest of the month, whole grains are advisable. Many people avoid beans because they make them feel gassy, but did you know that beans should be soaked prior to cooking? Traditionally, beans were soaked to make them more bioavailable and easier to digest, with limited side effects. Now we grab a can of beans and pour it in a dish without even rinsing it. Ideally beans should be soaked for certain lengths of time depending on the type of bean.

In Eastern medicine grains are considered heavy and sweet. These qualities lend themselves to tonifying the yin of the body, or structure and fluids, and also the spleen. Sometimes when yin is lacking in some way, shape, or form, we may crave sweet taste and baked goods. Sweet has the capacity to nourish and moisten, and if yin fluids are deficient then that's exactly what we need. Oftentimes yin deficiency means there is excess heat or inflammation somewhere in the system. This may also cause craving of sweet, especially if there is dryness in the mucosal linings of the body. If grains are being unnecessarily avoided, it could be a set-up for sweet cravings. When there are whole grains in the diet, the heaviness and sweetness of them tonifies or adds energy and nutrition to the spleen's vitality. When the spleen's vitality is not waning, it means that we have what we need to have, functioning well, to properly transform food and fluids. When the spleen's vitality is lacking, we may not be digesting or assimilating properly.

We also need salt in the diet to tonify the spleen vitality. Good salt like Himalayan pink salt is heavy and nourishing and helps support the root of vitality in the body—the kidneys. By tonifying the kidneys, we are supporting the spleen system that supports digestion. Because dinner will fall in kidney time according to the Eastern medicine circadian rhythm, or organ clock, eating foods that support the kidney system at that time is in harmony with our natural daily cycle. We can add some raw foods into the diet in the earlier part of the day, but doing so later or at night is not aligned with the energetics happening in the body at that time. During the day the energy of the body is moving up and out, and the yang qi or vitality of the body is at its strongest. It peaks at noon. This is why we are supposed to eat the most in the earlier part of the day, and have our largest meal when the sun is highest in the sky.

Just as the sun radiates heat and light most at this time, so does our interior. This makes it the perfect time to consume, impart nutrients, and transform, just as the radiation from the sun does in the strongest daylight hours. This is why we want to do the most active things earlier in the day, such as exercise and activate the digestion by actively putting food in our bodies, and then relying on the body to deal with it.

Just after the sun's peak in the early, yang part of the day, the more yin aspect of the day takes hold. Yin is still and deals with sustenance and stability. There is a heaviness and inward-moving energetic that predominates. When the body is most yin it needs us to back off so it can focus on more internal energetics that aren't so outwardly active.

Research shows it's better to eat during daylight hours, which indicates there is some flexibility in the summer months when it doesn't get dark until later. I recommend finishing the last meal before dusk. In most parts of the world in winter that will be a little earlier, and I think a realistic time for our modern lifestyle is between 5:00 and 6:00 p.m. In the summer it may be a bit later.

In the dark hours the body goes into scavenge and repair mode, and much of it is done as we sleep. By not actively instigating the beginning phases of the digestive process in the more yin part of the day, we are setting our bodies up to do what it needs to in the later hours, instead of carrying over more yang activities into the night when yin stillness is supposed to dominate.

This is why sleep habits and hygiene are so important. Hygieia, the

Greek goddess associated with healing, is recognized by her name, from which we get the word *hygiene*. But hygiene in the Greek sense wasn't just about washing hands and keeping the living space clean and orderly. It was, like diata, about living a healthy life and having daily habits that maintain health. Hygieia's father, Asklepios, the god of medicine, is the deity associated with healing when one is sick, but Hygieia is associated with how one stays well. We help ourselves stay well by living according to the natural impulse and rhythm in nature and within the body. We have become top-heavy with desire and wants, and it is time to come back to living in harmony with our entire selves and with nature. Following the natural rhythms of the external environment and internal ecosystem is how we do this. Sleep is part of it, as is preparing one's mind and body for sleep by living with wisdom throughout the day. Sometimes we just need to get out of the way. By doing so, the body's natural intelligence can take charge and we will start to feel better by default.

Daily Schedule

I find it works best to have an outline of how I'd like my day to go. Here is a general framework of the daily protocol:

Morning Routine
The first few minutes of your day can set the tone for the entire day.

- It is best to wake around dawn. Waking around 6:00 a.m., we are coming into consciousness while melatonin secretion is fading. This may mean we start the day slowly. This is okay.
- Begin with a routine that allows for gradual movement into the day, both mentally and physically. Sit up gently and take a few breaths.
- Consciously let the feet connect with the ground.
- Follow this with tongue scraping, teeth brushing, and elimination.
- Drink a cup of room temperature or warm or hot water with or without lemon, based upon how your stomach feels.

- Sit quietly for a few minutes and breathe. Use the breathing technique from the previous chapter.
- Take some time for mindful stillness. Allow the body and mind to come into sync with one another, making note of how you feel this day. Then allow yourself to connect with your inner sense or greater sense of self and well-being. The one that is there always, regardless of how you feel at any given moment. Let this aspect of awareness be your guiding force throughout the day.

Moving more actively into your day, this is a good time to journal. I like the morning pages that are taught in Julia Cameron's book, *The Artist's Way*. Take whatever time you have and just write, stream of consciousness, without regard for correct grammar, sentence structure, or thought completion. Just empty out the subconscious residue from the night and previous day. This is another great way to clear the *tamasic,* or dullness, cobwebs remaining after the night's sleep, and transition into a peaceful presence. This is also a good time to write contemplatively or meditate contemplatively. If there is something weighing heavily, after centering with the initial sitting and breathing and mindful syncing, use this time as an opportunity to let it shine. That may sound contrary to how heavy and dark things that weigh on us feel, but we need to bring them to the light to be observed and contemplated.

This contemplation is not consternation and overthinking. Rather, it is mindful awareness from a place of feeling centered to your best ability in the moment. It is a syncing of the mind and body in a different way, offering the opportunity to create space around an object of angst, which lacks space and makes you feel less light, spacious, and free. Suspend this issue in your mind's eye and allow yourself to feel it in your body. Where in your body do you feel it? What, if anything, does it feel similar to or remind you of? This thinking, like morning pages, is often nonlinear and may feel irrational. And it is! It is reason-based in that there is an intention to bring an issue into focus, but it is emotive in that it asks how the body is responding. This process deepens the resonance between mind and body so that there is an experience of being whole. The power in this alone allows for transformation because it requires a degree of letting go in order for it to happen. The letting go is in the willingness to shine light on what we perceive as darkness, which can take any form or be called by any name.

Once there is a sense of awareness of what the object of focus is, and how it feels in the body, there is the breath. Breathe deeply around the edges of the object and see how it feels inside, then create space around it with the breath, your inherent spaciousness. The edges will become more diffuse and the power of the object will wane. It may wax again if the mind sinks into being overcome by it, but this is a choice. It may be an unconscious one at first, but the more this process is practiced, the more conscious seemingly overbearing obstacles become, and the less automatic. By breathing spaciousness into something we feel stuck about and recognizing its resemblance to other situations or objects in life, we give it less and less power over us. It is then that we can realize we are in a place of stability and clarity to an extent we never thought possible.

Contemplating this way is a process. At the end of each individual session, allow yourself to be the parent in the situation and create a boundary with your intention that states the session is over for now, and the issue or object can be revisited later. This does not mean it is being suppressed, as you've consciously taken it out into the light of awareness. It simply means that you've created a healthy boundary for it and that the presence of it is not controlling your thoughts, feelings, or actions. Allow a sense of forgiveness, both of other and self, and breathe light and space into yourself. Reconnect with the awareness of an internal compass that is always there guiding you, even when you think you don't hear it, a sense of greater knowing and well-being that is the foundation of mind and body. It is your substrate of existence that is always okay, no matter what crisis, attachment, or aversion may arise. Abide in this for a moment.

An intentional yoga practice or other form of exercise is a great follow-up to this process. Going for a walk, taking deep breaths, or any kind of mild to moderate exercise is good now. Nothing too strenuous.

Next is dry brushing. Dry brushing can be done with a loofah, but I recommend Ayurvedic raw silk *garshana* gloves. These allow more fluidity in the process and feel more subtle and comfortable on the skin. Start with your toes and brush up to the groin. Then start at the finger tips and brush in toward the armpits. This stimulates lymphatic flow, the superficial circulation, and the immunity of the skin by stirring up the ecosystem of the skin. Next do circular motions on the joints and belly. Finish with your sides, and be gentle on the face and neck.

After dry brushing take a nice relaxing shower with natural products. Choose natural soaps with few additives or perfumes. After bathing use oils to soothe, moisturize, and protect the skin. People governed by air may use sesame blended with olive oil; those with excess heat can use coconut with olive oil; and those with healthy, well-nourished skin can use olive oil or some other blend. The same oils should be used on the face. Try out different oils and combinations and see which work best for you and your skin. Note that this may change seasonally or in response to how you feel on any given day. Natural, pure, cold-pressed oils not only nourish the skin, they feed the beneficial bacteria that live in and on it. Shampooing presents particular challenge for those who like to color their hair, because unless pure henna is used, dying the hair is not a natural process. The color process almost invariably involves chemicals, and almost all of the supporting products are not natural, because they're designed to keep color dye in your hair.

Breakfast

Breakfast can be either a hot grain cereal with seasoning, for example cinnamon or cardamom, and a little raw local honey or maple syrup, or you may want to have *kitchari,* a blend of split yellow mung beans and rice (see recipe on page 195). Another option is *congee,* an East Asian rice porridge (see recipe on page 197). If you are looking for an alternative to morning coffee, I suggest a barley drink or herbal tea. If you're still weaning off caffeine, some lightly steeped (a minute only) green tea is good. I also like peppermint tea, tulsi tea, or a pinch of cumin, coriander, and fennel steeped in hot water.

Digestive Stimulants

If you'd like to work on stimulating digestive fire, you could have a small cup of fresh ginger tea twenty minutes before meals, or a thin slice of ginger with a squeeze of lime juice, a sprinkle of Himalayan salt, and a drip of raw honey (eaten like a cracker). This is a natural perk-me-up for your digestive juices. If you prefer a pill or tablet, and have a phlegmy constitution, you may want to try the traditional Ayurvedic digestive aid *trikatu*. I also like Maharishi Ayurveda's Herbal Di-gest. It's a combination of the famous peppery, gingery digestive aid trikatu with other herbs and spices that help to perk up digestion, and it contains all the tastes. I recommend one to two of these right before or with breakfast, lunch, and dinner, but only while you're doing a dietary reset, experiencing sluggish digestion, gas, or bloating, or if having a large or heavy meal. Be sure to let the tablet sit on the tongue before swallowing so the taste of it can be experienced.

Between Meals

Cumin-coriander-fennel tea is lovely between meals. It's a digestive aid that helps to gently cleanse the GI tract, and helps prevent bloating and gas. It can easily be made at home by combining these three seeds and adding just a pinch to a cup of hot water. Let it steep a few minutes and sip on it between meals, or if you're experiencing cravings. It can be made stronger or weaker. Note that it is not a replacement for water consumption.

Water Consumption

Water consumption should be roughly half the body weight in ounces, and not cold or iced. If reflux is an issue, don't gulp, only sip. Around mealtimes, keep water consumption light so it doesn't interfere with digestion. When finished eating, the stomach should be about 80 percent full, or ⅓ fluids, ⅓ solids, and ⅓ empty. The fluids referred to are those in the meals we eat, not a glass of water as this may dilute digestive potency.

Let's Talk About Smoothies

There are no smoothies in the dietary reset, or as a regular staple in the diet when not doing the reset. If you're having digestive issues, a smoothie may make you feel lighter, but this may be because you aren't breaking down solids well, have slow gastric emptying, or some other reason that could be corrected with the right attention and protocol. Smoothies aren't recommended for several reasons: They mix together many things that ordinarily aren't combined; smoothies are cold, or have mostly cold, heavy ingredients; and most smoothies include some kind of processed powder. These may be okay here and there, but on a regular basis these powders are too dry and smoothies overall may be difficult to digest. They may go right through you without being properly assimilated. If stools are loose and the tongue has teeth marks on the edges, indicative of spleen qi deficiency, this is probably what is happening. There's no reason to tax the body with these if you have good digestion and are eating a well-rounded diet. It's not like smoothies are at the top of the list when it comes to what foods feel really nourishing and grounding to the body. You wouldn't eat your way through a trip to Italy by consuming smoothies, would you? Our bodies are worth more than that.

Lunch

Lunch should be the largest meal of the day, ideally between 10:00 a.m. and 1:00 p.m. During the dietary reset it will most likely be kitchari. On a regular basis, though, it should be your heaviest meal of the day, and also the time when you eat a salad, if you're having one that day.

Dinner

For dinner, if you're doing the dietary reset, you'll have kitchari again most likely. If not and it's a regular day, make this meal light. By that I mean easy to digest and assimilate. Have something brothy, or soup. Miso soup is great, as are many others. Some people get in the habit of having breakfast for dinner. Flip your meals around so you have something more substantial for breakfast, and a hot cereal or soupy congee for dinner. When not doing the dietary reset, allow yourself a little sweet for this meal, too.

Although eating leftovers is not recommended in Eastern teachings, sometimes you have to choose the lesser of two evils: Is it better to grab fast food or reheat a home-cooked organic meal? I choose the latter.

Evening Routine

The evening routine is rather important. It will be the most difficult aspect of the reset for most people for a number of reasons. Maybe you'll want to eat late with your spouse who doesn't get home till 9:00 p.m. Or you will need to cook two meals because the kids won't eat kitchari. You may want sugary snacks at night, or want to binge on potato chips. Or maybe you will want to binge watch your favorite show and not go to bed till 2:00 a.m., when your body should be detoxifying in the deepest part of the sleep cycle.

The evening may be a good time to prepare for the next day. Soak some beans or grains for breakfast. Try some forest bathing or take a soothing epsom salt bath. These practices are not only rejuvenating and healing, they are detoxifying and feel good. If you want to go the extra mile in your reset and really relax, and you don't have little ones tugging at you, enjoy self-oil massage before your bath. Some prefer to do this after dry brushing in the morning.

Self-oil massage aids in the circulation of the san jiao and rasa, or nutritive fluids, and stimulates lymphatic circulation, helping to release toxins. Another way it aids in toxin release is to bind to fat-soluble toxins in the skin and draw them out through the pores for elimination.

Self-oil massage is like a gentle hug for the nervous system. The oil enters the pores and hugs or calms the nerves. It's soothing, nourishing, and feeds the skin microbiome. Please note, if you're suffering from a skin rash, or an infection such as herpes, self-oil massage is temporarily contraindicated, as it may actually spread the pathogen.

Self-Oil Massage

- Start by heating a bottle of good quality oil in hot water in the sink. Olive oil is fine.
- Stand on a towel on the floor in a warm room and make sure you have something to put over you and the oil, because you'll be leaving it on for 15 to 20 minutes after you apply it fully.
- Just as with dry brushing, apply liberally in strokes toward the heart. Massage circles on the joints and abdomen. Do the face, scalp, and everywhere you can reach.
- Wrap up and either breathe, meditate, or read something inspirational.
- Then get in a hot bath or shower. Slough off the excess oil, but don't wash with soap. Just wash your hair if it needs it. Some people prefer to leave the oil on, or add castor oil or sesame oil to the scalp to nourish the hair overnight, then shower it out in the morning.

If you find yourself trying to stave off cravings, have a cup of cumin-coriander-fennel tea. Then before bed I suggest the Ayurvedic remedy triphala. I really like Maharishi Ayurveda's triphala formula because it includes cabbage rose, and so offers an even gentler effect on the system. Triphala is a wonderful remedy as it is useful for all body types, contains vitamins and minerals, and can be taken long term. It is comprised of three fruits that help to gently assist the body in its natural detoxification process: *amalaki* (Indian gooseberry), *bibitaki* (beleric, a tree fruit), and *haritaki* (a bitter tree fruit).

Try to be in bed by 10:00 p.m. Being in bed by ten, and asleep by then if possible, causes you to miss catching a second wind when transformation time rolls back around. This is the best time to rest, digest, and detox, not use mental functions or eat.

This is the protocol for the seven to ten days. Please factor in your exercise regime. In Eastern medicine just breaking a sweat is adequate, not dripping with sweat. This is because over-exercising can deplete fluids, blood, and vitality. Try to get a walk in every day, preferably in natural surroundings so there is an element of forest bathing present in your daily routine. If that isn't possible, remember to look up at the sky every so often. This elevates and clears the mind.

Metabolic Types and Food Choices

In chapter 3 I introduced the concept of metabolic types, and determining where you fall based on stool diagnosis. You can watch how things shift during the reset and make alterations to your veggies and to the consistency of your kitchari and/or congee accordingly. Remember that during the reset you will likely not be eating some of these foods. They may be incorporated afterward. For those eating congee at every meal during the reset, the foods listed below can help guide the selection of proteins to add.

Irregular/Dry Metabolism

Irregular or dry metabolism is associated with an increase of air element and potential stagnation in the flow of vitality. Conditions and foods that exacerbate these conditions are anything cold, light, dry, mobility promoting, and rough. As a basic rule, it is best to favor warm, cooked, grounding, and smoother foods and food preparations. For example, soups and stews are wonderful, and even better if pureed because the texture is smooth. Kitchari and congee are ideal. These types would also benefit from oils, so do add some high-quality extra virgin olive oil or ghee to each meal. Grounding foods include root vegetables and cooked whole grains. Cooking or stewing and adding a little spice to fruit is preferable over raw, and it is best to avoid dried fruits. Dry powders mixed into breakfast cereals or smoothies are also best avoided. Regardless of all this, the most important, and often the most difficult guideline for this metabolic type to implement is eating at regular meal times every day.

Here is a sample food list for those who experience irregular or dry digestion:

Almonds	Mung beans
Amaranth	Oats
Apricots	Oils (not processed vegetable oils)
Asparagus	Okra
Avocado	Papayas
Beef	Parsnip
Beets	Peanuts
Berries	Peas
Black olives	Pistachios
Butter	Plums
Buttermilk	Prunes
Carrots	Pumpkin seeds
Cherries	Quinoa
Dark meat	Rice
Dates	Salmon
Eggs	Sardines
Fennel	Sesame seeds
Figs	Shrimp
Flax	Squashes
Ghee	Sweet potatoes
Green beans	Tuna
Macadamia nuts	Walnuts
Mango	Watercress
Miso	Wheat

This is an abbreviated list; a more complete list can be found in *Handbook of Chinese Medicine and Ayurveda.*

Fast/Hot Metabolism

Those who experience faster metabolism with loose bowel movements may not be completely absorbing what they ingest because food is moving too quickly through them to be properly fermented. For these fast or hypermetabolic types, stools can be urgent, soft, loose, fall apart, burning, or liquidy/oily. They tend to have difficulty dealing with a lot of oils and greasy foods. Oil stokes fire, and fire is usually what is in excess in the digestive tract in these types. Basic recommendations include eating more cooling fresh foods such as fruits and vegetables, and staying well hydrated. Noticing what aggravates the mood and avoiding such triggers or creating ways of working with them so that they don't have such an impact on the gut is also important. Don't eat when frustrated. These types tend to have more difficulty with processing anything that will speed up their metabolism. This includes things that are hot, sharp, intense, oily/greasy, and light, so we want to favor things that have a cooling effect on the system. This doesn't mean iced products, but a cooling metabolic effect; there's a big difference. Iced beverages and foods can also contribute to too much cold in the system, further hampering the body's ability to fully assimilate what's being consumed. Sweet, cooling, soft, grounding and nourishing foods and fluids are best.

The food list for a faster, hot metabolism is as follows:

Adzuki beans	Cardamom
Apricots	Cauliflower
Asparagus	Celery
Avocado	Chicken
Barley	Chickpeas
Black beans	Cilantro
Broccoli	Coconut
Brussels sprouts	Coconut oil
Butter	Coriander
Cabbage	Cucumber

Dill	Rice
Flax	Saffron
Ghee	Spearmint
Leafy greens	Split peas
Lentils	Sprouts
Lettuce	Sunflower seeds
Lima beans	Sweet apples
Melon	Sweet berries
Milk	Sweet cherries
Mint	Sweet plums
Mung beans	Sweet potatoes
Oats	Turkey
Olive oil	Venison
Parsley	Watermelon
Pear	Wheat
Peas	Zucchini
Pumpkin	

Sluggish/Damp Metabolism

If you know you are prone to having more sluggish or slow digestion, you should definitely be exercising and making sure there is enough liquid in your diet, whether or not you are doing the reset. These bowel movements tend to be copious, large, sticky, heavy, sluggish, and pale. In the case of hypo- or slow, dull metabolism, we want to favor warm, pungent, and spicy foods. This metabolic type is more typical of a predominance of earth element. People experiencing hypometabolism may crave sweets because they lack vitality and have more difficulty digesting heavier foods and large quantities of grain. We need to perk things up in people who are experiencing hypometabolism. The afore-mentioned Maharishi Ayurveda supplement, Herbal Di-gest, is great for this, as is the standard Ayurvedic remedy trikatu, the three spices.

These types actually need more fermented foods than the other types, and may even wish to supplement with a probiotic during the dietary reset. They may also want to use a higher dal to rice ratio, and double the veggies added to the kitchari.

These types tend to run cool, heavy, and moist, so they need to counteract these tendencies with foods that are light, dry, and warming. These include:

All spices
Almond oil
Amaranth
Apples
Apricots
Asparagus
Barley
Beet
Black beans
Broccoli
Brussel sprouts
Cabbage
Cauliflower
Celery
Cherries
Chickpeas
Chilies
Cranberries
Eggs
Figs
Flax oil
Freshwater fish
Garlic

Leafy greens
Leeks
Lemon
Lentils
Lettuce
Lima beans
Lime
Millet
Mung beans
Navy beans
Onion
Peach
Pear
Peppers
Pomegranate
Prune
Quinoa
Radish
Raspberry
Safflower oil
Spinach
Venison
White meat poultry

Kitchari and Congee

In Eastern medicine some version of a porridge, soup, or congee is recommended in times of illness, fatigue, or recovery from traumatic life events. These preparations include well-cooked, nutritious ingredients that are easy to digest. The idea behind eating simply at these times is to give the body something basic so it can do what it needs to heal. These simple gruels are also useful at times to simplify the diet or do a gentle cleanse. They allow the body to use energy normally spent digesting more complicated foods to instead heal and detoxify the deeper tissues, while also meeting basic nutritional needs so the body has the strength it needs to detox and heal.

The primary recipe I recommend comes from my own experience using kitchari in seasonal cleansing, get-well meals, and dietary reset regimens. This dish consists primarily of a legume called *moong* (mung) *dal* and either white basmati or sona massori rice. Right now, those of you who are thinking you need a FODMAP diet or are on an anticarb mission may be turned off by the sound of this. I can promise you that in most situations this meal, when consumed one to three times a day for seven days or more, can help ease digestive woes of many descriptions and even help with weight loss. I've experienced it and have seen it over and over again with my clients.

Let's dissect the dish. Moong dal, or mung beans, are an excellent source of protein, fiber, vitamins, and minerals.[2] Split yellow mung beans can be purchased at most health food stores or online, and in my opinion are a superfood we would all do well to incorporate into our diets. They're easy to digest and are the one bean that doesn't cause gas or bloating.[3] When combined with white basmati rice they have a very low glycemic load.[4] This makes them an excellent choice for people concerned with blood-sugar balance. In fact, kitchari is recognized for its ability to help regulate blood sugar, and mung beans have been shown to have a protective effect in animal studies when blood sugar spikes.[5] For those concerned with cholesterol levels, there is even evidence they may help inhibit LDL cholesterol oxidation.[6] Mung beans also balance cytokine release, thereby reducing potential for inflammation, and contribute to the activation of cholecystokinin (CCK) that helps us to feel full.[7] During a cleanse, digestion may slow once we have eliminated foods that have been used as crutches to speed transit time, for example caffeine, alcohol, raw foods, and chilies, so we need to consume something that is easily assimilable. Kitchari is the perfect food for this.

ࣷ Kitchari Recipe

Serves 2–3

4–5 cups water

¼ cup split yellow mung beans

¼ cup basmati or sona masoori rice

¹/₈ teaspoon turmeric

¼ teaspoon cumin seed

¹/₈ teaspoon yellow mustard seed

¹/₈ tsp ground fenugreek

¼ teaspoon fresh ginger

Salt and pepper to taste

Vegetables of choice

Extra virgin olive oil or ghee to taste,
   more or less based on metabolic type

To prepare kitchari, start by soaking the split yellow mung beans in water for an hour or two. Then drain the beans, add the rice, and rinse together several times. I use about half mung beans and half rice. If you want a really sweet, almost buttery kitchari, soak the mung beans with the rice for two hours before rinsing and cooking. Bring them to a boil, then turn it to a simmer. Add some turmeric, cumin seed, fresh ground ginger, salt, mustard seed, and whatever other spice you like to the simmering mixture. When the kitchari is almost done cooking, which will vary in time depending on whether you presoaked it or not, you can add your chosen vegetables to it, or cook them separately on the side—lightly sautéed on medium heat in a good quality olive oil or ghee, or roasted in the oven. A dollop of ghee on kitchari can be heavenly. I prefer Pure Indian Food's Cultured Ghee, or make my own.

The kitchari can be modified so that there are more mung beans, more rice, or more or less water depending upon desired consistency. I recommend you play with different recipes and adjust the consistency to determine what you like best at what time of day.

If you're unable to eat mung beans or have an aversion to kitchari, you can use congee instead. Or you may choose to eat both kitchari and congee during your digestive and dietary reset.

Congee is an East Asian rice porridge dish that is nutritious and easy to digest. It tonifies the spleen qi and builds blood and yin. It is soothing, light, and delicious. Often eaten for breakfast, it is also a wonderful medicinal dish for rebuilding strength during and after illness or injury; it doesn't tax the digestion or the body's resources at such a delicate time. Congee is eaten to ease constipation and diarrhea, soothe an inflamed digestive tract, and boost milk production in nursing mothers. During stressful times it can be eaten at any time of day in place of more complicated meals to simplify the daily routine and ease digestion. It's easy to make and can be tweaked in innumerable ways to accommodate one's needs. Although short grain rice is usually recommended, any rice may be used—brown or white—and vegetables or protein sources added. The spices and consistency may also be adjusted. The ratio of rice to water is anywhere from 1:5 to 1:10.

✑ Congee Recipe

Servings vary based on consistency—about 3 when prepared on the thicker side

½–1 cup rice, preferably short grain

5–10 cups water or broth, depending on desired consistency

1 teaspoon grated ginger

Vegetables of choice (spinach, celery, fresh corn, cabbage, leek, turnips, and bok choy are nice additions)

Salt and pepper to taste

Extra virgin olive oil or ghee to taste, more or less based on metabolic type

Rinse the rice a few times and add the desired amount of fluid to the pot. Bring to a boil then reduce to low heat and cover most of the way. Add ginger and vegetables and remember to stir occasionally as it may stick to the bottom of the pot. Cook times will vary depending on type of rice, just keep an eye on it. It usually takes about an hour. It is finished when the rice looks broken apart and the texture looks silky and soupy. Season to taste with salt and pepper and extra virgin olive oil or ghee.

For choosing vegetables in the congee and kitchari, I usually encourage a visit to the local farmer's market and a chat with the farmers. See what's in season and what is calling to you, even if you don't know what it is. The farmers can tell you how best to prepare what may be unfamiliar. Since you probably aren't making huge, varied meals at this time, it should be fairly easy to learn about new veggies. You may prefer to have a food list that specifies which veggies to choose for the reset, and later, what foods to choose in general. My primary recommendation is that you listen to what you feel most drawn to. If certain foods are calling to you, there may be a reason for that. Your own intuition is more important than any food list anyone can give you. For those still having difficulty deciding, look to your poop for guidance.

In chapter 3 we discussed the metabolic types and stool analysis. This is where that information comes in handy. I recommend you go back and look at that chapter again. As you begin the reset, your bowel habits may begin to change. Usually they will become more formed, regular, and only once or twice a day if they were previously loose and more frequent, and they may even float more. For some people they will slow down. They may change consistency from little pebbles to something more substantial, but the transit time may slow. If this is the case, reflect on what you think could have been causing you to poop more before the reset. Did your body rely on caffeine every morning? Lots of raw veggies? It can take weeks to reset the digestive rhythm after years of caffeine reliance. This can be an uncomfortable time. If you find that you are really uncomfortable and are going for days without pooping, I recommend eating some dates, figs, or prunes after dinner. You can also take a good quality probiotic during the reset. Try substituting brown rice for white, as it contains more fiber. If this doesn't help, you could try some tea containing senna, or the Maharishi Ayurveda Herbal Cleanse supplement. This is a nicely balanced formula that isn't harsh on the system, but does the trick. Please note, senna is habit-forming and products that contain it should be used only when absolutely necessary and not on a regular basis.

Reset Recap

Four days to two weeks prior to the start of the reset, do the temporary elimination regimen, eliminating:

Caffeine	Meat
Alcohol	Dairy
Processed food	Eggs*
Refined sugar	Nuts and seeds
Refined flour	Hot spices

---

*Eggs are included in the reset only for those eating strictly congee for more than three days.

Daily Schedule

Wake by 7:00 a.m. at the latest.

Be mindful of initial thoughts, feelings, sensations, and movement.

Scrape the tongue.

Brush the teeth.

Evacuate the bowels.

Drink warm or room temperature water, which may contain lemon.

Meditate/breathe/journal (or you may prefer to do this after dry brush and shower).

Dry brush.

Shower.

Eat breakfast.

Drink coriander-cumin-fennel tea between meals along with adequate water.

Twenty minutes before lunch, take two Herbal Di-gest tablets, or a small slice of ginger with a sprinkle of Himalayan salt, a squeeze of lime juice, and a drop of honey.

Eat lunch by 1:00 p.m.

Drink coriander-cumin-fennel tea and adequate water.

Again, twenty minutes before your next meal take one or two Herbal Di-gests, or a small slice of ginger with Himalayan salt, lime juice, and a drop of honey.

Eat dinner by 5:00 p.m.

In the evening relax, go for a walk, read, meditate, journal, bathe, self-massage.

Take triphala before bed.

Go to sleep by 10:00 p.m.

That's it. Just watch your bowel habits and make adjustments as needed. After the seven days, begin to reintroduce more foods. Start with something you're questioning. Let's say it's gluten or dairy, then for one meal add that back in first. Maybe you can make a risotto with cheese and rice. Or if it's gluten that worries you, have some seitan or a whole grain containing gluten, like barley. See how you feel doing that for a couple of days. If you feel reactive, make note of it. Give yourself some more time without it and reintroduce something else. If it's fine, add something else. Maybe it's alcohol or meat. Start with smaller portions of meat.

Many chronic coffee drinkers actually don't want it again, not right away, and usually cave out of familiarity or ritual more than craving. Most don't go back to it as a regular staple in the diet. Sweet foods taste really sweet, and that sensitivity lends itself to less consumption of sweets in the long run. Eat out, see how you feel. If your digestion feels off afterward, do a meal of kitchari to give it a rest and recoup.

Here are some tips to remember. Wheat and gluten-containing whole grains are a primary source of dietary fiber, particularly the insoluble kind. This is the kind that not only adds bulk and helps scrape the excess gunk from the GI tract, but can also speed motility and feeds the good bacteria in the gut. These grains are widely available in Western culture and for all of these reasons it is best not to avoid them if you don't need to. A client of mine who has celiac disease told me the one thing she would do if she could is to tell everyone worried about gluten intolerance to revisit this belief and work on tonifying their digestion instead of eliminating these grains.

Avoid iced food and drinks and any food in excess. Do not overeat or undereat, and don't eat when stressed, angry, or upset. I recommend soaking beans before consumption, and rinsing them well if canned. Wash your fruit and veggies before cutting or biting into them. Favor organic whenever possible. I look to a Mediterranean diet or blue zone diet as a good model for long-term microbial and digestive well-being. Blue zone diets tend to be more omnivorous and are rich in a variety of fruits and vegetables, with a higher consumption of fruits, veggies, and whole grains mixed with meats and oils, and most likely result in greater microbial diversity as a result of their variation, fiber heaviness, and naturally fermented food products.

Hopefully you now have a fuller understanding of what to eat and when to eat it, as you follow the best guidance of all—that which comes from your body. Here is a handy summary of the general Eastern medicine food-consumption guidelines:

- Stick to mostly cooked foods.
- Front-end most of the food you eat to the early part of the day.
- Avoid iced foods and drinks; even in summer, have them in moderation.
- Calm down or center before eating if you're upset.
- Eat whole, organic, unprocessed food whenever possible.
- Eat whole fruits and veggies, including the skins where appropriate, instead of juicing.
- Try to incorporate as many tastes as you can into each meal.
- Recognize that yogurt is a condiment or small side dish, not an entrée.
- Have salads or raw vegetables when the sun is high and digestive fire is the strongest.
- Leave at least four hours between meals.
- Wait until the stomach is empty before snacking.
- Don't drink coffee on an empty stomach.

These guidelines are recommended regardless of metabolic or mind-body constitutional type.

If it's too much to commit to a dietary reset program, commit to something you can start. Maybe it's eating each of the tastes in every meal (see the box on page 130), establishing a daily routine, going to bed earlier, exercising, decreasing caffeine intake, or reducing cold or iced food and beverages. Many people have fast-paced lives and little kids or are retired and busier than they were when they worked. Remember the importance of having balance in life. That includes not suddenly overdoing it in the self-care department, as that is rarely sustainable. Start small and allow new, more healthful habits to unfold gradually.

Find what brings you joy and do it regularly. Breathe. Stop eating by 6:00 p.m. and go to bed by 10:00 p.m. These are great places to start. Or maybe you can incorporate some time in nature, whether a walk, a swim, or just a sit on the ground with a good book or scenery to admire. Do this for all of you: mind, body, microbiome, and spirit. And always remember, you are (literally) not alone.

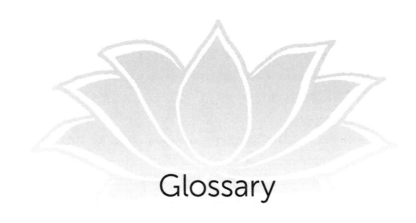

Glossary

agni: Metabolic heat, digestive fire in Ayurvedic medicine; transforms raw materials into nourishment and nutrition.

anabolic: Tissue-building metabolic activity.

Bacteroides: Bacteria type usually found in abundance in those eating diets high in animal products and low in fiber. Associated with increased secondary bile acid production, inflammation, and, as a result, higher risk of gastrointestinal disease.

biofilm: Substance secreted by colonies of microbes that encloses them and serves as a protective sheath.

butyrate: Short chain fatty acid (SCFA) associated with inflammatory regulation and primary food source for gut epithelial cells.

catabolic: Tissue-degrading metabolic activity.

catecholamine: Type of neurotransmitter.

chong mai: Chinese medicine term for the storage vessel for qi and blood.

chyme: Partially digested foodstuffs.

cold: One of the six pathogenic factors, or pernicious influences, in Chinese medicine that may cause disease.

commensal: A long-term biological interaction in which one organism or species benefits while the other has a neutral reaction.

congee: East Asian rice porridge.

Corynebacterium: Beneficial axillary microbe that works with the body to maintain or restore balance, is also present in the vagina and fights off pathogens.

dal: Dried, split pulses.

damp: One of the six pathogenic factors, or pernicious influences, in Chinese medicine that may cause disease.

defensive qi: Immune vitality; also called wei qi.

deficiency: A lack of substance or functioning.

dinacharya: Daily routine one is recommended to follow in Ayurveda.

dosha: Type of mind-body structure and energy. Technically, dosha means "imbalance" and refers mostly to bodily types; there are three dosha types in Ayurveda—vata, pitta, and kapha.

dryness: One of the six pathogenic factors, or pernicious influences, in Chinese medicine and a quality of vata dosha in Ayurveda.

dysbiosis: An imbalance or malfunction in the microbiome of an individual.

ekadashi: *Ekadashi,* which means "eleven," is the eleventh day after the full and new moons, when some Hindus refrain from eating grains.

elements: The five building blocks of matter and how nature manifests and behaves.

enteric: Pertaining to the intestines.

enterotype: Constitutional type based upon which bacterial types are dominant in the gut microbiome.

evil qi: The umbrella term for the six pathogenic factors, or pernicious influences, of Chinese medicine; may refer to any one of them.

excess: Too much of a substance or a buildup of it where it doesn't belong.

exposome: The cloud of chemicals and microbes we emit and breathe in.

functional medicine: A branch of modern medicine that has a more holistic framework and tries to address the root cause of disease.

garshana: Dry brushing.

he-sea point: Acupuncture channel points located around the knees and elbows. These points are located on the twelve regular channels and address the qi as it moves deeper and more powerfully through the body. They are often used to strengthen the earth element, or spleen and stomach, and to nourish the water element.

heat: One of the six pathogenic factors, or pernicious influences, in Chinese medicine that may cause disease.

interstitium: Fluid-filled space between tissues, lined with connective tissue; correlates with the san jiao of Chinese medicine.

jin ye: Body fluids in Chinese medicine; synonymous with *rasa* in Ayurveda.

kapha: A humor in Ayurveda, one of the three doshas, made up of water and earth elements and associated with mucus.

kitchari: Indian dish made with mung beans and rice.

Lactobacillus: Beneficial bacteria found to largely colonize and maintain the health of the vagina, parts of the gut, and breast tissue.

limbic: System in the brain that deals with emotion and memory.

macromolecules: Carbohydrates, lipids, and proteins.

mesentery: Organ that surrounds the intestines and anchors them within the abdominal cavity, protecting nerves and blood vessels during movement; correlates with the mo yuan/membrane source in Chinese medicine.

mesoderm: Middle layer in early embryonic development.

microbiota: The entire collection of microbial communities that contribute to the composition of a living being: anything that's alive.

mo yuan: In Chinese medicine, "membrane source," correlates to the mesentery organ.

mucoid plaques: Believed by some to be a sticky or membranous substance that adheres to the intestinal walls; may be made up of microbial biofilms.

mucosa: Mucous membrane.

munda agni: Dulled, sluggish digestion or metabolism.

mycobiome: Part of the microbiota made up of yeasts and fungi.

omentum: Fatty tissue sheath covering the abdominal organs.

peristalsis: Involuntary wavelike muscle contraction and relaxation that pushes food through the GI tract.

pitta: A humor in Ayurveda, one of the three doshas, made up of fire and water and deals with heat, metabolism, and transformation.

po: One of the five spirits in Chinese medicine, po is anchored in the lung tissue.

postbiotic: Supplement containing bacterially derived compounds or metabolites.

prebiotic: Supplement containing food for gut microbes.

Prevotella: Bacterial type that is associated with carbohydrate consumption (thus often dominant in vegans). Ferments dietary fiber into short chain fatty acids that may reduce inflammation.

probiotic: Supplement containing beneficial microbes.

psychobiotic: Pre- and probiotic supplement filled with microbes found to positively influence gut-brain communication.

purgation: Therapeutic modality of evacuating the bowels.

qi: Vitality. The energetics, magnetics, ionic charges, and radiation circulated throughout, emitting from, and animating the individual, which includes some aspects of the microbiome.

qigong: Gentle breathing and movement exercises that cultivate vitality.

rasa: In Sanskrit, "enjoyment." In Ayurveda, bodily fluid, also the word used for taste.

ritucharya: Seasonal routine in Ayurveda.

Saccharomyces boulardii: Mycobiome species used in probiotics to decrease diarrhea and crowd out an overgrowth of candida (a yeast in the microbiome that often overgrows in the absence of beneficial microbes to keep it in check, thereby becoming pathogenic).

sama agni: Balanced digestion.

san jiao: Triple warmer, or three environments organ in Chinese medicine; correlates to the interstitium.

scleroderma: Autoimmune condition that causes unnecessary tissue scarring.

serosa: Outer lining of the intestines.

shaoyang: The hinge between the interior and exterior levels of the body in Chinese medicine.

shen: Spirit, mind, or consciousness in Chinese medicine; may refer to the collective five shen (wu shen) or to the shen of the heart.

submucosa: Layer of the GI tract that surrounds the mucosa and is made of connective tissue containing lymph and nerves.

summerheat: One of the six pathogenic factors, or pernicious influences, in Chinese medicine.

swara: System of yoga focused on nostril breathing and how it affects physiology and mental states.

symbiosis: Occurs when one or two organisms or groups living in close proximity benefit from one another.

t'ai chi: Chinese internal martial art.

tenesmus: Continuous urge for a bowel movement.

tikshna agni: Hypermetabolism; quick, hot digestion.

tonify: To support or add to.

transcutaneous: Through the skin.

tridosha: The three humors of Ayurveda.

turbinates: Ridges in the nose made of erectile tissue.

Vaastu: The art of placement in India, similar to the Feng Shui of China.

vata: One of the three humors in Ayurveda associated with mobility, cold, and dryness.

villi: Fingerlike projections that line the intestinal tract and increase surface area, allowing for greater nutrient absorption.

virome: The sum total of viruses that make up the microbiota.

vishama agni: Irregular, dry metabolism or digestion.

wei qi: Immune vitality; also called defensive qi.

wind: One of the six pathogenic factors, or pernicious influences, of Chinese medicine.

wu shen: The five spirits or aspects of consciousness in Chinese medicine.

yang: The source physiological heat and energy that the body needs to survive. If yin is matter, yang is energy.

yin: The opposite of yang. In Taoist cosmology, the feminine, receptive principle of nature, and the structure and fluids of the body in Chinese medicine.

Notes

Introduction. The Fascinating World of Microbes

1. Montgomery and Biklé, *Hidden Half of Nature,* 37.

2. Montgomery and Biklé, 24.

3. Montgomery and Biklé, 25.

4. Montgomery and Biklé, 27.

5. Yong, *I Contain Multitudes,* 10.

6. Das et al., "Concept of Krimi," 57–69.

7. Montgomery and Biklé, *Hidden Half of Nature,* 27.

8. Yong, *I Contain Multitudes,* 11–12.

9. Yong, 19.

10. Mayer, *Mind-Gut Connection,* 25.

11. Yong, *I Contain Multitudes,* 44.

12. Yong, 230.

Chapter 1. Everything but the Kitchen Sink

1. Yong, *I Contain Multitudes,* 61.

2. Belizário, "Human Microbiomes," 1050.

3. Wikipedia, "Mycobiome," accessed January 4, 2019.

4. David Pride and Chandrabali Ghose, "Meet the Trillions of Viruses that Make Up Your Virone," The Conversation (webpage), October 9, 2018.

5. Grice and Segre, "Skin Microbiome," 244–53.

6. Grice and Segre, 244–53.

7. Grice and Segre, 244–53.

8. Hamblin, "1,458 Bacteria Species."

9. Hamblin.

10. Ossolo, "Antiperspirants, Deodorants."

11. Blakemore, "Armpit Transplants."

12. Blakemore.

13. Rutsch, "Meet the Bacteria."

14. Rutsch.

15. Steven Lin, "Is Your Mouth Microbiome More Important than Your Gut?" MindBodyGreen (webpage), accessed February 5, 2020.

16. Mark Burhenne, D.D.S., "The Oral Microbiome & Its Impact on Every Other System in the Body," Ask the Dentist (webpage), updated February 6, 2020.

17. Mark Burhenne, D.D.S.

18. Steven Lin, "Is Your Mouth Microbiome More Important than Your Gut?" MindBodyGreen (webpage), accessed February 5, 2020.

19. "Gum Disease Linked to Alzheimer's, Study Claims." Analysis by Bazian, NHS.UK (webpage), January 24, 2019.

20. Ruth Williams, "Booger Bacteria's Sweet Immune Suppression," The Scientist (webpage), September 6, 2017.

21. Williams.

22. National Institutes of Health, "Eye Microbiome Trains Immune Cells to Fend Off Pathogens in Mice," NIH (webpage) News Release, July 11, 2017.

23. Olivia Willis, "Why Your Vaginal Microbiome (Like Your Gut) Is Important," Australian Broadcasting Corporation (webpage) Health News, November 21, 2017.

24. Willis.

25. Willis.

26. Willis.

27. Baker, Chase, and Herbst-Kralovetz, "Uterine Microbiota."

28. American Microbiome Institute, "What Happens If You Give C-Section Babies a Vaginal Microbiome?" *Microbiome Institute* (blog), February 8, 2016.

29. American Microbiome Institute.

30. Zimmer, "Germs in Your Gut."

31. Zimmer.

32. Olivia Willis, "New 'Bladder Microbiome' Discovery Could Change the Way we Treat UTIs," Australian Broadcasting Corporation (webpage) Health News, June 2, 2018.

33. Rachael Rettner, "Men's Testes Have a 'Microbiome.' Could It Affect Fertility?" Live Science (webpage), June 19, 2018.

34. Rettner.

35. Kara Gavin, "Bacteria in Your Lungs? New Microbiome Study Shows How They Get There," M Health Lab, *Lab Report* (blog), February 24, 2017.

36. Gavin.

37. Gavin.

38. O'Dwyer, Dickson, and Moore, "Lung Microbiome," 4839–47.

39. Mueller et al., "Infant Microbiome Development," 109–17.

40. Mueller et al.

Chapter 2. The Kitchen Sink

1. "Digestive System: Histology of the Alimentary Canal," Anatomy and Physiology (webpage), January 9, 2014.

2. "Digestive System."

3. Vighi et al., "Allergy and the Gastrointestinal System," 3–6.

4. Junger, *Clean Gut,* 33.

5. Junger, 26.

6. Lu et al., "Extraoral Bitter Taste Receptors," 181–97.

7. International Foundation for Gastrointestinal Disorders, "Disorders of the Small Intestine," About GI Motility (webpage), last updated March 24, 2016.

8. John Easton, "Specific Bacteria in the Small Intestine Are Crucial for Fat Absorption," UChicagoMedicine (webpage), April 11, 2018.

9. Easton.

10. Easton.

11. Easton.

12. Enders, *Gut,* 45.

13. Jill Corleone, "Are Bananas High in Soluble Fiber?" SFGate (webpage), November 27, 2018.

14. Liu et al., "Butyrate," 21–29.

15. Liu et al., 21–29.

16. Buck, *Acupuncture and Chinese Medicine,* 286.

17. Liu, "Butyrate," 21–29.

18. Jill Corleone, "Are Bananas High in Soluble Fiber?" SFGate (webpage), November 27, 2018.

19. Liu et al., "Butyrate," 21–29.

20. Elizabeth Rajan, M.D., "Digestion, How Long Does It Take?, Mayo Clinic (webpage), December 31, 2019.
21. Enders, *Gut,* 47.

Chapter 3. Quite Simply, Poop

1. Tungland, *Human Microbiota,* 399.
2. "Cow Dung Uses and Used for Centuries," *TrueAyurveda* (blog), September 4, 2014.
3. Rajeswari, Poongothai, and Hemalatha, "Antimicrobial Activities of Cow Dung."
4. Liji Thomas, M.D., "History of Fecal Transplant," News Medical (webpage), last updated August 23, 2018.
5. Eakin, "The Excrement Experiment."
6. "Anatomy and Normal Microbiota of the Digestive System," Lumen Learning, Microbiology (webpage), accessed February 18, 2019.
7. Montgomery and Biklé, *Hidden Half of Nature,* 31.
8. "About the Rome Foundation," Rome Foundation (webpage), accessed March 22, 2019.
9. Kunal Ahuja, and Kritika Mamtani, "Probiotics Market Size by Ingredients," Global Market Insights (webpage), November 2019.
10. Montgomery and Biklé, *Hidden Half of Nature,* 30.
11. Bollinger et al., "Human Secretory Immunoglobin A."
12. Montgomery and Biklé, *Hidden Half of Nature,* 31.
13. Velasquez-Manoff, "Western Diet."
14. Jeff Leach, "East African Hunter-Gatherer Research Suggests the Human Microbiome is an Ecological Disaster Zone," The Conversation (webpage), February 28, 2017.
15. Leach.
16. Leach.
17. Schorr et al., "Gut Microbiome of the Hadza."

Chapter 4. Making Connections

1. Biologydictionary.net, "Mesentery," May 13, 2018.
2. Carina Wolff, "The Scientist Who Discovered A New Organ—The Mesentery—A Year Later," Simplemost (webpage), March 22, 2018.
3. Wolff.

4. Editors of Encyclopaedia Britannica, "Mesoderm," Encyclopaedia Britannica (webpage), July 20, 1998.

5. "Mesenchymal Stem Cells: The 'Other' Bone Marrow Stem Cells," EuroStemCell (webpage), accessed April 1, 2019.

6. Online Etymology Dictionary, "Mesentery."

7. Rivera et al., "The Mesentery, Systemic Inflammation, and Crohn's."

8. Rivera et al.

9. Rivera et al.

10. Rivera et al.

11. Rivera et al.

12. Macpherson and Smith, "Mesenteric Lymph Nodes," 497–500.

13. Guarino, "Meet the Mesentery."

14. Chang et al., "Cutting Edge," 4361–65.

15. "Da Yuan Yin," TCM Cure (webpage), November 15, 2006, http://cm-cure .com/Da-Yuan-Yin-Chinese-medicine-herbal-formula.

16. "Da Yuan Yin."

17. "Da Yuan Yin."

18. "Da Yuan Yin."

19. "Cao Guo," American Dragon (webpage), accessed June 5, 2017.

20. "Da Yuan Yin," TCM Cure (webpage), November 15, 2006, http://cm-cure .com/Da-Yuan-Yin-Chinese-medicine-herbal-formula.

21. "Da Yuan Yin."

22. "Da Yuan Yin."

23. "Da Yuan Yin."

24. "Da Yuan Yin."

25. "Da Yuan Yin."

26. Rachael Rettner, "Meet Your Interstitium, a Newfound 'Organ,'" LiveScience (webpage), March 27, 2018.

27. Deadman, *Manual of Acupuncture,* 153.

28. Deadman, 154.

Chapter 5. Mind Your Microbiome

1. Office of Dietary Supplements. "Vitamin D: Factsheet for Health Professionals," National Institutes of Health (webpage), updated August 7, 2019.

2. Brad Yantzer, "D-I-E-T, The Four-Letter Word," *TrueAyurveda* (blog), April 15, 2019.

3. Manning, *Against the Grain,* 176.

4. Philip Perry, "Scientists are Zeroing In on Where Intuition Comes from, Biologically," BigThink (webpage), January 29, 2018.

5. Valerie van Mulukom, "Is it Rational to Trust Your Gut Feelings? A Neuroscientist Explains," The Conversation (webpage), May 16, 2018.

6. Sarkar et al., "Psychobiotics."

7. Sarkar et al.

8. Richard Conniff, "Take a Deep Breath and Say Hi to Your Exposome," Scientific American (webpage), September 28, 2018.

9. Rogers et al., "Gut Dysbiosis to Altered Brain Function."

10. Rogers et al.

11. Ye and Liddle, "106 Gastrointestinal Hormones and the Gut Connectome."

12. Ye and Liddle.

13. Bergland, "Tranquility Promotes Healthier Microbiome and Gut-Brain Axis."

14. Rogers et al., "Gut Dysbiosis to Altered Brain Function."

15. Rogers et al.

16. Ye and Liddle, "106 Gastrointestinal Hormones."

17. Bergland, "Tranquility Promotes Healthier Microbiome."

18. Mayer, *Mind Gut Connection,* 25.

19. Bercik, et al., "Intestinal Microbiota."

20. Bob Quinn, with Erin Moreland, "Gu Syndrome: An In Depth Interview with Heiner Fruehauf," ClassicalChineseMedicine.org (webpage), 2008.

21. Philip Perry, "Scientists Are Zeroing In on Where Intuition Comes from, Biologically," BigThink (webpage), January 29, 2018.

22. Perry.

23. Yong, *I Contain Multitudes,* 257–58.

24. Twohig-Bennet and Jones, "Health Benefits," 628–37.

25. Twohig-Bennett and Jones.

26. Clemens G. Arvay, MSc, "How Being in the Forest Actually Boosts Immunity, According to Science." MindBodyGreen (webpage), accessed April 24, 2019.

Chapter 6. Food for Vitalizing Mind and Body

1. Psomagen, Terms of Service," Psomagen.com (webpage), updated November 1, 2019.

2. Psomagen.

3. National Human Genome Research Institute (NHGRI), "Genetic Discrimination," US NIH (webpage), accessed May 17, 2019.

4. Wikipedia, "Olestra," accessed April 26, 2019.
5. Melissa Kravitz, "6 Foods that Are Legal in the U.S. but Banned in Other Countries," Business Insider (webpage), March 1, 2017.
6. Kravitz.
7. Kravitz.
8. "Azodicarbonamide (ADA) Frequently Asked Questions." US FDA (webpage), accessed April 26, 2019.
9. Fallon and Enig, *Nourishing Traditions,* 133.
10. Menni et al., "Omega-3 Fatty Acids Correlate with Gut Microbiome Diversity."
11. Joseph Mercola, "Canola Oil Proven to Destroy Your Body and Mind," Mercola (webpage), December 27, 2017.
12. Mercola.
13. Mercola.
14. Yong, *I Contain Multitudes,* 54.
15. Montgomery and Biklé, *Hidden Half of Nature,* 5.
16. Montgomery and Biklé, 55.

Chapter 7. Change Your Life, Change Your Microbiome

1. Smolinska et al., "Volatile Metabolites in Breath," 1–11.
2. Maciocia, *Foundations of Chinese Medicine,* 196–97.
3. Marcus Woo, "Body Maps Expose the Chemical Residue that Coats Our Skin," Wired (webpage), March 30, 2015.
4. Woo.
5. "Chronobiology: The Science of Time," Chronobiology (webpage), accessed May 4, 2019.
6. "Chronobiology"
7. John Douillard, "Seasonal Living: The Original Biohack," LifeSpa (webpage), March 14, 2019.
8. John Douillard, "3-Season Diet Challenge," LifeSpa (webpage), accessed Feb 6, 2020.
9. Kevin Jiang, "Bacterial Circadian Clocks Set by Metabolism, Not Light." U Chicago News (webpage), December 15, 2015.
10. Chappell, "Nobel Prize in Medicine."
11. Chappell.
12. Wehr, "Melatonin and Seasonal Rhythms."
13. Wehr.

14. "Melatonin: The Sleep Hormone That Provides a Good Sleep," BrainEffect (webpage), accessed May 11, 2019.

15. Roizen, Crupain, and Spiker, *What to Eat When,* 32.

16. Roizen Crupain, and Spiker, 34–35.

17. Roizen, Crupain, and Spiker, 33–35.

18. Roizen, Crupain, and Spiker, 29.

19. Roizen, Crupain, and Spiker, 30.

20. "Melatonin: The Sleep Hormone That Provides a Good Sleep," BrainEffect (webpage), accessed May 11, 2019.

21. Michael J. Breus, "Unlocking the Sleep-Gut Connection," Psychology Today (webpage), January 8, 2016.

22. Michael Breus, "The Latest on Sleep and Gut Health," The Sleep Doctor (webpage), May 29, 2018.

Chapter 8. Dietary Reset Protocol

1. Junger, *Clean Gut,* 127.

2. "Mung Beans, Mature Seeds, Cooked, Boiled, without Salt, Nutrition Facts & Calories," SelfNutritionData (webpage), accessed May 22, 2019.

3. John Douillard, "Get to Know the Kitchari Cleansing Bean." LifeSpa (webpage), September 15, 2015.

4. Douillard, "Get to Know the Kitchari Cleansing Bean."

5. Douillard, "Get to Know the Kitchari Cleansing Bean."

6. Chung et al., "Protective Effects of Organic Solvent Fractions."

7. Douillard, "Get to Know the Kitchari Cleansing Bean."

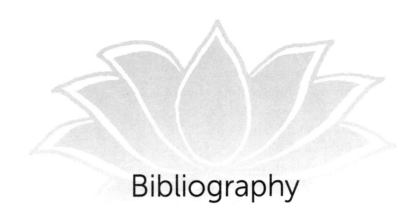

Bibliography

Baker, James M., Dana M. Chase, and Melissa M. Herbst-Kralovetz. "Uterine Microbiota: Residents, Tourists, or Invaders?" *Frontiers in Immunology* 9 (2018): 208.

Belizário, Jose E., and Mauro Napolitano. "Human Microbiomes and Their Roles in Dysbiosis, Common Diseases, and Novel Therapeutic Approaches." *Frontiers in Microbiology* 6 (2015): 1050.

Bercik, P., E. Denou, J. Collins, W. Jackson, J. Lu, J. Jury, Y. Deng, et al. "The Intestinal Microbiota Affect Central Levels of Brain-Derived Neurotropic Factor and Behavior in Mice." *Gastroenterology* 141, no. 2 (2011): 599–609.

Bergland, Christopher. "Tranquility Promotes Healthier Microbiome and Gut-Brain Axis." *Psychology Today,* January 7, 2016.

Blakemore, Erin. "Armpit Transplants Could Make You Less Stinky." *Popular Science,* February 2, 2018.

Bollinger, R. Randall, Mary Lou Everett, Daniel Palestrant, Stephanie D. Love, Shu S. Lin, and William Parker. "Human Secretory Immunoglobin A May Contribute to Biofilm Formation in the Gut." *Immunology* 109, no. 4 (2003): 580–87.

Buck, Charles. *Acupuncture and Chinese Medicine: Roots of Modern Practice.* Philadelphia: Singing Dragon, 2014.

Cameron, Julia. *The Artist's Way: A Spiritual Path to Higher Creativity.* Los Angeles: Jeremy Tarcher/Perigee, 1992.

Chang, Sun-Young, Hye-Ran Cha, Osamu Igarashi, Paul D. Rennert, Adrien Kissenpfennig, Bernard Malissen, Masanobu Nanno, Hiroshi Kiyono, and

Mi-Na Kweon. "Cutting Edge: Langerin+ Dendritic Cells in the Mesenteric Lymph Node Set the Stage for Skin and Gut Immune System Cross-Talk." *Journal of Immunology* 180 (2008): 4361–65.

Chappell, Bill. "Nobel Prize in Medicine Is Awarded to 3 Americans for Work on Circadian Rhythm." NPR, October 2, 2017.

Chung, Ill-Min, Min-A Yeo, Sun-Jim Kim, and Hyung-In Moon. "Protective Effects of Organic Solvent Fractions from the Seeds of *Vigna radiata* L. Wilczek against Antioxidant Mechanisms." *Human and Experimental Toxicology* 30, no. 8 (2011): 904–9.

Das, Jeuti Rani, Hermanta Bikash Das, Sisir Kumar Mandal, and Surendra Kumar Sharma. "Concept of Krimi in Perspective of Modern Era: A Review." *Journal of Ayurveda and Holistic Medicine* 3 (2015): 57–69.

Deadman, Peter, and Mazin Al-Khafaji, with Kevin Baker. *A Manual of Acupuncture.* Sussex, UK: Journal of Chinese Medicine Publications, 1998.

Douillard, John. *Eat Wheat: A Scientifically and Clinically-Proven Approach to Safely Bringing Wheat and Dairy Back into Your Diet.* New York: Morgan James Publishing, 2017.

Eakin, Emily. "The Excrement Experiment: Treating Disease with Fecal Implants." *The New Yorker,* November 24, 2014.

Enders, Giulia. *Gut: The Inside Story of Our Body's Most Underrated Organ.* Vancouver, BC: Greystone Books, 2015.

Fallon, Sally, and Mary G. Enig. *Nourishing Traditions: The Cookbook That Challenges Politically Correct Nutrition and Diet Dictocrats.* Washington, DC: New Trends Publishing, 1999.

Gomez, Carine, and Pascal Chamez. "The Lung Microbiome: The Perfect Culprit for COPD Exacerbations?" *European Respiratory Journal* 47 (2016): 1034–36.

Grice, Elizabeth A., and Julia A. Segre. "The Skin Microbiome." *Nature Reviews Microbiology* 9, no. 4 (2011): 244–53.

Guarino, Ben. "Meet the Mesentery: Irish Scientists Say This Gut Membrane Should Be Upgraded to an Organ." *Washington Post,* January 4, 2017, Morning Mix.

Hamblin, James. "1,458 Bacteria Species 'New to Science' Found in Our Belly Buttons." *The Atlantic,* December 18, 2012.

Johari, Harish. *Ayurvedic Healing Cuisine: 200 Vegetarian Recipes for Health, Balance, and Longevity.* Rochester, Vt.: Healing Arts Press, 2000.

Junger, Alejandro. *Clean Gut: The Breakthrough Plan for Eliminating the Root Cause of Disease and Revolutionizing Your Health.* New York: HarperOne, 2013.

Ling Shu Jing. *Spiritual Axis.* Translated by Giovanni Maciocia. Honolulu: University of Hawaii Press, 1993.

Liu, Ji Hu, Ji Wang, Ting He, Sage Becker, Guolong Zhang, Defa Li, and Xi Ma. "Butyrate: A Double-Edged Sword For Health?" *Advances in Nutrition* 9, no. 1 (2018): 21–29.

Lu, Ping, Cheng-Hai Zhang, Lawrence Lifshitz, and Ronghua ZhuGe, "Extraoral Bitter Taste Receptors in Health and Disease." *Rockefeller University Press Journal of General Physiology* 149, no. 2 (2017): 181–97.

Maciocia, Giovanni. *The Foundations of Chinese Medicine: A Comprehensive Text for Acupuncturists and Herbalists.* Elsevier Limited: London, 2005.

Macpherson, Andrew J., and Karen Smith. "Mesenteric Lymph Nodes at the Center of Immune Anatomy." *Journal of Experimental Medicine* 203, no. 3 (2006): 497–500.

Manning, Richard. *Against the Grain: How Agriculture Has Hijacked Civilization.* New York: North Point Press, 2004.

Mayer, Emeran, M.D. *The Mind-Gut Connection: How the Hidden Conversation within Our Bodies Impacts Our Mood, Our Choices, and Our Overall Health.* New York: Harper Collins, 2016.

Menni, Cristina, Jonas Zierer, Tess Pallister, Matthew A. Jackson, Tao Long, Robert P. Mohney, Claire J. Steves, Tim D. Spector, and Ana M. Valdes. "Omega-3 Fatty Acids Correlate with Gut Microbiome Diversity and Production of N-carbamylglutamate in Middle Aged and Elderly Women." *Scientific Reports* 7, article no. 11079 (2017).

Metsovas, Stella. *Wild Mediterranean: The Age-Old, Science-New Plan for a Healthy Gut with Food You Can Trust.* Avery, N.Y.: Pam Krauss/Avery, 2017.

Montgomery, David, and Anne Biklé. *The Hidden Half of Nature: The Microbial Roots of Life and Health.* New York: W.W. Norton and Company, Inc., 2016.

Mueller, Noel T., E. Bakacs, J. Combellick, Z. Grigoryan, and M.G. Dominguez-Bello. "The Infant Microbiome Development: Mom Matters." *Trends in Molecular Medicine* 21, no. 2 (2015): 109–17.

O'Dwyer, David N., Robert P. Dickson, and Bethany B. Moore. "The Lung Microbiome, Immunity, and the Pathogenesis of Chronic Lung Disease." *Journal of Immunology* 196, no. 12 (2016): 4839–47.

Ossolo, Alexandra. "Antiperspirants, Deodorants Change Your Armpit Microbiome." *Popular Science,* February 4, 2016.

Rajeswari, S., E. Poongothai, and N. Hemalatha. "Antimicrobial Activities of Cow Dung Extracts against Human Pathogens." *International Journal of Current Pharmaceutical Research* 8, no. 4 (2016): 9–12.

Rivera, Edgardo D., John Calvin Coffey, Dara Walsh, and Eli D. Ehrenpreis. "The Mesentery, Systemic Inflammation, and Crohn's Disease." *Inflammatory Bowel Diseases* 25, no. 2 (2019): 226–34.

Rogers, G. B., G. B. D. Keating, R. Young, M-L Wong, J. Licinio, and S. Wesselingh. "From Gut Dysbiosis to Altered Brain Function and Mental Illness: Mechanisms and Pathways." *Molecular Psychiatry* 21 (2016): 738–48.

Roizen, Michael F., Michael Crupain, and Ted Spiker. *What to Eat When: A Strategic Plan to Improve Your Health and Life through Food.* Washington, DC: National Geographic, 2018.

Rutsch, Poncie. "Meet the Bacteria That Make a Stink in Your Pits." NPR, March 31, 2015.

Sarkar, Amar, Soili Lehto, Siobhan Harty, Timothy Dinan, John Cryan, and Phillip Burnet. "Psychobiotics and the Manipulation of Bacteria-Gut-Brain Signals." *Trends in Neurosciences* 39, no. 11 (2016): 763–81.

Schorr, Stephanie L., Marco Candela, Simone Rampelli, Manuela Centanni, Clarissa Consolandi, Giulia Basaglia, Silvia Turrone, et al. "Gut Microbiome of the Hazdza Hunter Gatherers." *Nature Communications* 5 (2014): 3654.

Smolinska, Agnieszka, Danyta Tedjo, Lionel Blanchet, Alexander Bodelier, Marieke J. Pierik, Ad A. M. Masclee, Jan Dallinga, et. al. "Volatile Metabolites in Breath Strongly Correlate with Gut Microbiome in CD Patients." *Analytica Chimica Acta* 1025 (2018): 1–11.

Tungland, Bryan. *Human Microbiota in Health and Disease: From Pathogenesis to Therapy.* Cambridge, Mass.: Academic Press, 2018.

Twohig-Bennett, Caoimhe, and Andy Jones. "The Health Benefits of the Great Outdoors: A Systematic Review and Meta-analysis of Greenspace Exposure and Health Outcomes." *Environmental Research* 166 (2018): 628–37.

Velasquez-Manoff, Moises. "How the Western Diet Has Derailed Our Evolution." *Nautilus* 030 (November 12, 2015).

Vighi, G., F. Marcucci, L. Sensi, G. Di Cara, and F. Frati. "Allergy and the Gastrointestinal System." *Clinical and Experimental Immunology* 153 (2008): 3–6.

Wang, Ju-Yi, and Jason Robertson. *Applied Channel Theory in Chinese Medicine: Wang Ju-Yi's Lectures on Channel Therapeutics.* Seattle, Wash.: Eastland Press, 2008.

Wehr, Thomas A. "Melatonin and Seasonal Rhythms." *Journal of Biological Rhythms* 12 (1997): 518–27.

Ye, Lihua, and Rodger A. Liddle. "106 Gastrointestinal Hormones and the Gut Connectome." *Current Opinion in Diabetes, Endocrinology, and Obesity* 24, no. 1 (2017) 9–14.

Yong, Ed. *I Contain Multitudes: The Microbes Within Us and a Grander View of Life.* New York: Harper Collins, 2016.

Zimmer, Carl. "Germs in Your Gut Are Talking to Your Brain, Scientists Want to Know What They're Saying." *New York Times,* January 28, 2019.

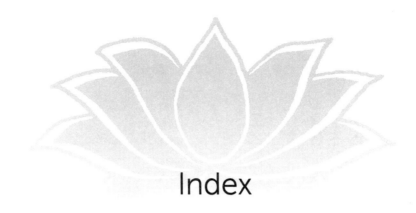

Index

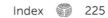